White Nights and Ascending Shadows

Jesse G. Monteagudo

White Nights and Ascending Shadows

An Oral History of the San Francisco AIDS Epidemic

Benjamin Heim Shepard

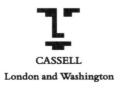

CASSELL

London and Washington

For a catalogue of related titles
in our Sexual Politics/Global Issues list
please write to us at an address below:

Cassell
Wellington House
125 Strand
London WC2R 0BB

PO Box 605
Herndon
VA 20172

First published 1997

British Library Cataloguing in Publication Data
A catalogue record for this book is available from the British Library.

Library of Congress Cataloging-in-Publication Data
Shepard, Benjamin Heim.
   White nights and ascending shadows: an oral history of the San
Francisco AIDS epidemic / by Benjamin Heim Shepard.
      p. cm.
   Includes bibliographical references and index.
   ISBN 0–304–70125–4 (hardback). — ISBN 0–304–70126–2
(paperback)
      1. AIDS (Disease)—California—San Francisco—History. I. Title
RA644.A25S45 1997
362.1'969792'0092279461—dc21   97–6629
                                                               CIP

ISBN 0 304 70125 4 (hardback)
      0 304 70126 2 (paperback)

"Maria" by Benjamin Heim Shepard first appeared in the *Antioch Review*,
Vol. 53, No. 2 (Spring 1995). Copyright ©1995 by the Antioch Review,
Inc. Reprinted by permission of the editors.

Typeset by Ben Cracknell Studios
Printed and bound in Great Britain by Creative Print and Design
(Wales), Ebbw Vale

Contents

Acknowledgements

Books aren't so much created as assembled from previously existing components and, in this case, memories. From the very beginning this book was about capturing a few of the *zeitgeistal* winds blowing through the San Francisco streets. It could only be done because a large number of people took part in the assembling process, sharing stories, expertise and references with me. I cannot preach enough about the communal spirit of assistance and civic pride displayed by the citizens of the Baghdad by the Bay who, when confronted with the opportunity to contribute to the public record a small piece of their extraordinary history, were more than happy to oblige. Countless unsuspecting individuals, named and unnamed, who came across my path over the last four years were asked to put in sweat equity in the construction process of this manuscript.

The book, of course, began with the Shanti Project. Hugo Manzo and countless others from the building first demonstrated the potential of the story and its applications. I am indebted to him and many others. Jim Snively, my very rigorous manager, deserves astounding credit for his lenience in allowing these conversations to continue and continue. Ramone Matos must be credited for suggesting I place ads calling for interviews in the local rags and providing me with a number of names of colleagues to call for assistance on the project.

The first step in the project of the book involved construction of questions to ask interviewees. David Boyer must be credited for input into the first list of questions, design of the flyer calling for interviewees, and countless referrals to other resource people including Bill Hayes of the San Francisco AIDS Foundation who also helped edit the questions. Boyer, as my roommate and fellow AIDS Inc.-er, council and ear, which I bent at will, deserves a great deal of credit.

Once the proposal was in place, Kurt Berrie, Derrick Burten, Brian Caulker, James Bristol, and Prof. Pastora San Juan Cafferty, my University of Chicago mentor, put a great deal of assistance into its polishing. Thanks are also due to Chicago's Tom D'Aunno, William Borden and Bertram Cohler. The biggest thanks go to Dan Volger for his professional marketing advice and his wonderful interview. Sara Brown's BUILD workshops and editorial assistance helped a great deal, as did Judith Types.

Numerous individuals helped to draw the attention of potential interviewees. Richard Chavez provided space in the Shanti Bulletin for calls for interviewees and gave me one of my best early interviews. Rebecca Denison, of WORLD, provided me with access to the newsletter, her offices, and the women of her organization. Nadine Lurie, of ACT UP Golden Gate, put me in contact with some of the group's finest minds.

Chris Culwell of *BAR*, Rebecca Paoletti, then of *SOMA*, and Larry Smith, then of *Media File Journal*, all deserve great thanks for their faith and encouragement by publishing the first glimpses of this work and the thought that lay behind it in their local pages. On the national scene, Robert Fogerty of *Antioch Review* and Jeffrey Williams of the *Minnesota Review* deserve thanks for their publication of an untried talent. Williams, in particular, through his constructive input about how to present this material, helped move the work out of a dead end. I thank Robert Fogerty for permission to use "Maria".

Professor Peter Nardi, of Pitzer College, who provided sound counsel all through this process, deserves a great deal of credit. The San Francisco Holocaust Oral History project provided me with a format, release, and guidelines for conducting oral history in the city. Dr. Ray Buchanan first served as historical mentor and tour guide of the age of anxiety years back.

My photographers showed a dynamic determination to tell this story. With little to go on but faith, Kelli Yon dedicated Saturday after Saturday journeying to photograph the city's underworld. And to Jake Peters I cannot give enough thanks for his contribution.

Then there were the friends, Megan Conroy, Marla Perez, and James Rogers, who provided a bastion of sanity, companionship and fun during years of absurdity and more than our fair share of drama in the city. Gerd Grace stuck with me through a move, two summers' worth of ridiculous behavior, late dinners, and anxieties around a never-ending manuscript. I am indebted to her.

My family provided the greatest moral support for the entire four-year saga of this project. Reverend Jack Shepard, Dad, dusted off his editing skills and put in "100 billable hours" hacking through the work. Professor Dorothy Shepard put in edit after edit on the proposal and manuscript. Without her polishing, the book might not have been able to fly. Jenn Shepard served as professional sound board and advisor in terms of a view of the publishing world.

And, of course, oral history does not happen without interviewees. To folks such as Robert Boulanget, who told me the story of his two lovers twice because once I lost the tape, I owe the most thanks. It takes an extraordinary kind of courage to tell one's life story to a complete stranger. I am truly indebted to Cleve Jones, who shared a significant piece of his public record. Nothing I can say accurately represents the level of respect I have for the courage and dignity the people with AIDS of San Francisco have brought to bear in persevering during plague time. Through their compassion for the ill among them, they have taught America that the sanctity of love transcends the story of a city and its ongoing struggle against misunderstanding.

B.H.S.

For the hope that one day America will shed its selective compassion for the ill and the dead in its midst.

Introduction

From Munich to Castro Street

"It's very frustrating because here I am at the pinnacle of my career. I could do literally anything I wanted in the world of journalism, and you're left with the strange feeling that your life is somehow finished without being completed," said Randy Shilts, author of the magnum opus of the AIDS pandemic, *And the Band Played On*, months before he himself died of AIDS in 1994 ("Randy Shilts," 1994). Activists, city officials, old friends and colleagues converged in droves at Glide Memorial United Methodist Church in San Francisco's decaying Tenderloin District the morning of February 22, 1994, to pay homage.

"Can an aging faggot get a seat around here?" John Cailleau, a Shilts acquaintance from the decadent '70s heyday, asked a guard.

"We don't use that word around here," the guard responded.

"A lot has changed since California Hall [San Francisco's Stonewall]," Cailleau thought to himself. Earlier in the week the Rev. Fred Phelps had announced he was bringing members of his Topeka, Kansas congregation to picket "the faggot writer['s]" funeral. Fears of violence lingered as the crowd of two thousand waited for the service to begin. Two men held signs, "OUR RIGHT TO LOVE" and "OUR RIGHT TO GRIEVE." In the end, the Phelps group was pelted with eggs and ran. Phelps tried to take refuge in a police van but the cops kicked him out (Raine and Flinn, 1994). The spectacle around the funeral encapsulated many things Shilts had fought for. All his life he had aspired for gays and lesbians to live and die with dignity and respect. Perhaps the most disturbing aspect of Shilts' death was the books he did not get to write, the memories lost. He was planning on writing his memoirs of San Francisco in the '70s, '80s, and '90s. This story, like those of so many others, is gone.

Waves

Randy Shilts wrote of the migration of a group to San Francisco and the destiny that befell those people. People flock to San Francisco in waves.

They always have. They come to find something which has eluded them within their lives. They come here to get away from the formality of the East Coast. This is the myth of San Francisco. Every year another wave. A couple of years ago, one-third of the graduating class from Brown University moved to San Francisco. Herbert Ashberry (1933:1) cites the Gold Rush of 1849 as the focussing event in the development of San Francisco's reputation as safe haven for America's outcasts:

> If the precious yellow metal hadn't been discovered in the auriferous sands of the Sacremento Valley, the development of San Francisco's underworld in all likelihood would have proceeded according to the traditional pattern and would have been indistinguishable from that of any other large American city. Instead, owing almost entirely to the influx of gold-seekers and the horde of gamblers, thieves, harlots, politicians and other felonious parasites who battened upon them, there arose a unique criminal district that for almost seventy years was the scene of more viciousness and depravity, but which possessed more glamour, than any other area of vice and iniquity on the American continent.

And waves continued. By 1941, soldiers came to ship off to fight the Japanese. Those who were discharged because of sexual orientation stayed. They certainly weren't going home to Altoona, Pennsylvania, to explain just exactly why they were not fighting the Good War. Shilts (1982: 50–1) elaborates on the war's social impact and role in the creation of a gay settlement in San Francisco. "Men were uprooted from generations-old family centers, pulled outside the ken of their peers' values . . . The military speeded up San Francisco's growth into a gay center." In the 1950s they came to North Beach for the poetry, the jazz, to get away from "Ozzie and Harriet" (a TV show), McCarthy and generational conformity. In the late '60s, they came to the Haight/Ashbury district for the acid, the Dead, the surreal, and as Robert Crumb confessed, "Some of that free love action." By the '70s, crowds in lumberjack shirts, jeans and hiking boots, with toned bodies and bar mustaches came for a piece of liberation and God knows what else on Castro Street. As the '80s turned into the '90s, another wave hit. The San Francisco Model was heralded around the world for an enlightened range of programs servicing people with AIDS. This time folks came to descend on San Francisco from all parts, ironically, for just a bit of that sanity, again hoping to heal themselves (Weiners, 1995).

Fading voices and memories

Across the city on the morning of Shilts' funeral, George hobbled with his walker out of an elevator at the AIDS housing facility where he lives and I work. He had wasted to a point where his emaciated bicep could be held between a thumb and forefinger. His once black mustache was now gray. His Creole accent was still thick.

"Hi Ben," he said as he sat on a couch in the lobby.

"How was the movie last night, George?" I asked.

"Pure camp," George smiled, "but I couldn't enjoy it too much because the seat was so uncomfortable. My rump's gotten so small, it's all bone. I don't get padding," George confessed. He died a month later. His old lover, Rick, came by the building to pack his things.

"After three days on the respirator, he told the doctor to pull the plug. He died within the night. The man never hurt a soul," Rick recalled.

"Except for the homophobes who came to the Stud in the '70s looking for fights. George told me he would prance around until one of them would start something then he'd beat the tar out of the guy."

"Yeah, he used to call home and tell me, 'I did it again. Now everyone in the bar is buying me drinks.' When he was done with one of those guys he would tell him, 'Go home and tell your friends you got beat up by a fag!'" Of the migrants who came in the '70s, the Stonewall Generation, a majority of them have passed. Their deaths leave a huge void.

Many of the PWAs (People with AIDS) where I work have told me they intended someday to write down everything they have learned. Melvin, a black man who served in the army in the Czech Sudetenland, told me stories about his years romping around Europe. He regretted not having written his story down. "I wanted the world to know that as a gay black man with AIDS, I have been able to make it." Sigemund, a blond-haired painter who walked with a limp, used to hobble through the building clad in dirty sweat pants, dress shoes, plus wire-rimmed glasses. He tried to hunt and peck his way through his memoirs before he became too suicidal to work. I found him odd looking until I saw one of his works at a local gallery. I saw in the brush strokes in his self-portrait the motion of his limp. It occurred to me that in the portrait as in his life, Sigemund's limp obfuscated the dignity of his face. The opportunistic infections eventually caught up with him and he died while seizuring.

These men lived through the litany of failures as doctors developed treatments with the sophistication of blood-letting; as Shilts (1987: 595) noted, the President shook his fist at "the Evil Empire" while failing even to mutter the word AIDS for six years and the plague raged unchecked. Having felt the consequences of our culture's awkward and frequently Byzantine means of grappling with death and disease, their time ran out; their experiences, for the most part, are lost.

The day Melvin died, I went to buy a tape machine to use for taping the recollections of other PWAs so as never to watch another story like his vanish. I made a flyer with the headlines: "Calling All Stories, Remember Reagan and GRID? Living Long Term with HIV?" and placed it all over the city. Although few women or people of color responded, gay men responded in force (Shepard, 1996). As PWAs willing to share the memories of the last twenty-five years are a difficult group to attract, I engaged in a form of snowball sampling, asking interviewees if they knew anyone else willing to talk, taking their names down and contacting them (Rubin and Babbie, 1993). I formally interviewed some thirty PWAs for the project.

Sometimes my position as an advocate is apparent. It is true, I feel passionately about issues where ignorance, selective compassion and cultural arrogance made life unnecessarily difficult for people already ill, postures which continue to impede a rational and humane policy toward putting a stop to the epidemic to this day.

But in my advocacy I can only make common cause. I am not HIV-positive. My life and my plans have never been impeded by it. I'd like to think of all Americans on Martin Luther King's terms, "We are bound together in a single garment of destiny" (Braithwaite and Lythcott, 1991). There are, however, limits to walking in other people's shoes.

Foundations

In an article titled, "Eros and Anxiety in *Fin de Siècle* San Francisco," I first interviewed PWAs about their lives in the context of the *fin de siècle* (Morten, 1979). The comparisons to the decadence of Vienna and Weimar, Germany are compelling. Inflation plagued both Carter and Hindenburg. Liberalism eros and suspicion of something sinister walked hand in hand in both eras. These premonitions came to fruition both in the '30s in Germany and in the '80s here. A culprit lay in the murky San Francisco fog just as Peter Lorre hid in the dark alley nights of Fritz Lang's 1931 psychological mystery *M*. Light bends (Williams, 1968). Weimar introduced the twentieth century to the idea of moral relativity (Gay, 1968; Kaes *et al.*, 1994; Derfler, 1990; Willet, 1978). The AIDS era offered the century its culmination.

AIDS in San Francisco grew out of the best, the most joyous decade in Gay History, the 1970s. The decade ended with assassins' bullets and riots much as in 1968 and '69. Photographs of Bobby Kennedy and Harvey Milk hung adjacent to each other in Hank Wilson's office in the Ambassador Hotel. The 1979 White Night Riots presented gays defending themselves and the end of the liberation decade with tooth and nail, a last stand, as if they knew something terrible was right around the corner, just as Fritz Lang, Oscar Kokoschka and Max Beckman knew a menace was in their presence during the Weimar years of the 1920s and '30s (Shilts, 1982; Johanns, 1992; Weitman, 1992).

The AIDS era in America followed the Vietnam era of the '60s and '70s, just as the country was trying to put the conflict behind it. The apparently unwinnable battle against the disease has been called the 1990s' Vietnam (Null, 1995). Tim O'Brien (1994) writes about Vietnam as a cancer he carries through his life. The Vietnam he speaks of applies to the malignant legacy this conflict has left on the American psyche. Through the Vietnam Syndrome, Americans acknowledge that awkward part of our ambiguous national identity which sees the world in terms of us and them and values human life with conditional love. Human lives become expendable. Stalin once claimed fifty deaths were tragedy, one million were politics. Through the story of HIV, we revisit these themes. Dr. Anthony Fauci of the National Institute of Health compares the daily rates of new infection to three 747s crashing a day. The UN stipulates the number is around 7500 a day (Simmons, 1995).

"The shadow of this country is coming through," Richard Chavez observed of the unending years of the epidemic. The 1979 White Night Riots unfolded because Supervisor Milk, "Mayor of Castro Street," as Shilts dubbed him, and Mayor Moscone were forsaken by a jury. Their assassin received a seven-year sentence for their murder. Message: it was all right for a former policeman to gun down a "faggot supervisor" (Shilts, 1982). It's OK for faggots in San Francisco to die by the thousands. America's selective compassion for the dead is the "Ascending Shadow" referred to in the title, *White Nights and Ascending Shadows*. Milk and Moscone were the first to be forsaken. Over the following eighteen years, 15,590 San Franciscans would die of the deadly plague while no national strategy was drawn to take on the epidemic (Kreigler, 1996). The White Night Riots cast a long shadow on the AIDS era. The riots continue to this day, a ghost dance. Interviewees recall that night and its legacy on the epidemic and the rest of their lives.

5

Contexts and attrition rates

The influence of disease on human history cannot be underestimated (Swenson, 1988; McNeill, 1976). Renaissances have been born out of plagues (Hartt, 1987). Early in 1995, Frank Rich wrote of the influence AIDS has had on our culture: "History may show that the epidemic has changed our culture in much the way that the cataclysmic carnage of World War I transformed English literature. However it turns out, this is the story of our time." AIDS has produced a generation of HIV-positive writers devoted to Sartre's idea of engagement, telling this story with their last gasps. Both Paul Monette and David Feinberg, who wrote books on AIDS themes, died in 1995. Writer Larry Kramer, who first recognized the impending disaster by founding GMHC (Gay Men's Health Crisis) and ACT UP (Aids Coalition To Unleash Power), is positive. Through her newsletter and organization, *WORLD*, Rebecca Denison does more for HIV-positive women than all S.F. AIDS Inc. combined. She is positive. Many of the most effective AIDS activists who have fought the pandemic the longest, are positive. They are lions in winter. The attrition rate is phenomenal.

In a final interview, Monette spoke of the responsibility of his HIV-negative colleagues, "We have to count on them to make sure our story is told and not forgotten. It's going to be a long time before history can look back and say, 'Oh, what was AIDS?'" (Zachary, 1995).

Methods: oral history and narrative approaches

I was able to interview a few such San Francisco lions, most notably Cleve Jones, as well as thirty other veterans of the epidemic. With a nod to Studs Terkel's (1967) methodology, I did not seek out those who already have forums for their ideas, instead leaning toward attempting to create a people's history of this epidemic. Jones, a noted exception, as the city's most famous street activist, offered the historical backbone which other personal histories flesh out.

As a social worker moonlighting as a social historian, I was interested in both listening to people tell their stories and tapping into social history. Consequently, the work utilizes contemporary narrative approaches as they overlap with oral history (Plummer, 1983; Sherman and Reid, 1994; Reisman, 1993; Martin, 1996). In so doing, I sought to ask each interviewee his or her life story (an approach sometimes called the humanistic or human sciences approach; see Plummer, 1983, and Cohler, 1994), placing the narratives within a context of the larger history of the AIDS epidemic in San Francisco.

White Nights and Ascending Shadows is a montage of life story interviews with thirty PWAs. The interviews function as a group to tell the oral history of a period, San Francisco from 1968 to 1995. The power of the work lies in the composition of interviews forming the story of the '70s migration to San Francisco, the election of the nation's first openly gay official, his assassination, the onset of a disease, and its impact on a city. The transcripts, although edited, cut, and pasted in the same format as Stein and Plimpton's (1982) *Edie: An American Biography*, are presented with an effort at maintaining the integrity of the interviews.

The interviews were conducted using a set list of questions, although most interviewees talked without interruption in accordance with both narrative and oral history methods utilized by the Holocaust Oral History Project. They emphasize that the interviewer has a list of questions to ask, but not to interrupt the interviewee's thought progression. Reisman (1993: 3) argues that narrative interviews produce results unique to qualitative research methods in the respect that:

> Respondents (if not interrupted with standardized questions) will hold the floor for lengthy turns and sometimes organize replies into long stories. Traditional approaches to qualitative analysis often fracture these texts in the service of interpretation . . . They eliminate the sequential and structural features that characterize narrative accounts.

My interviewees tended to answer most of the questions I intended to ask anyway within their narratives. If certain points were not covered, I would go back and ask for more information. Through open-ended questions, allowing the real story within the story to come out, the migration to San Francisco and the context of the Gay Liberation Movement found its way into the narrative. These stories are, in turn, presented through a thematic narrative.

Starting with Thomas and Znaniecki's (1918–19) *Polish Peasant*, social researchers have used life stories to analyze the subjective meaning of social life. Chicago sociologist Clifford Shaw, one of the field's innovators, stipulates: "The life-history record is a relatively new instrument for the study of human behavior" (1931: ix). Oral traditions, however, have been used to recount the shape and history of time, forming world views of cultures, nations, and peoples (Martin, 1995: 4).

Cohler (1994) emphasizes that the life story account can provide insight into the depth of a social condition. He argues that in

the study of lives in disorder, such as resulting from the impact of poverty and psychiatric illness, the human science is the most appropriate mode for understudying development and social change as forces impacting the study of lives over time. The human science perspective is the foundation of inquiry regarding both personal development and such directed intervention as psychotherapy and community intervention.

Sherman and Reid (1994: 286–328) highlight the use of qualitative research in policy and program evaluation. As such, this work utilizes narratives to assess and evaluate AIDS policy in San Francisco.

Despite the debates about the relative merit of statistical vs. case studies and life histories (McNight, 1987; Kurtz, 1984: 85–6), narrative approaches have received renewed interest in recent years (Martin, 1996). Kelley (1995: 351) explains that qualitative case studies better fit the spirit of postmodern narrative approaches than do controlled experimental design studies. They strive to understand world views rather than measure them. Realities are not considered fixed.

Martin (1995) has attempted to integrate social work and oral history on the basis of: a) obtaining information where little evidence exists or where documentation is suspect; b) revising history in which conclusions are suspect; c) protecting against loss of history; and d) collecting data to paint a holistic picture of biopsychosocial functioning.

Freedman and Combs (1996: 1) use the metaphor of the life story to consider "people's lives as stories." The narrative life story telling process allows people to rebuild and remember previously dislocated aspects of their lives into whole forward leaning units (Borden, 1992: 136). The narrative account allows us to watch the mysterious thought process of development as the individual places the tragedies, joys, and traumas of his or her life into context. To the extent that people's lives are stories, the narrative approach is perfect for use with those suffering from disease for it integrates and highlights internal thought and spirit with the external reality of the individual, whose body may be failing.

As life histories represent narrative truths, they do not always represent historical truth. Narrative approaches emphasize the subjective account. I do not vouch for facts stated by interviewees or suggest these accounts represent everyone. Borden (1992) writes, "Each person becomes a historian of the self, developing an internally consistent interpretation of the life cycle so that past, present, and future are experienced as congruent." The work does not, however, serve, as Schlesinger (1996) warns, to use history as a form of political therapy.

As the twentieth century lurches toward culmination, oral tradition fades, and quite unsurprisingly, people wander lost within dark woods, hidden from themselves and their communities. Many narrative theorists approach the field from a postmodernist point of view which acknowledges the existence of social constructs and a monolithic dominant culture. Freedman and Combs (1996: 1) use the metaphor to refer to the idea: "Every person's social, interpersonal reality has been constructed through interaction with other human beings and human institutions." This dominant culture, against which all points of view are measured, is perceived as a source of the modern demoralization (Kierkegaard, 1859: 85). It produces a reifying, flattening out of personal memory and heritage (Marcuse, 1977, 1964; Freedman and Combs, 1996: 26–7). Marcuse (1977: 73) stipulates: "All reification is forgetting." Oral tradition offers us a way out of the forest.

In striving to compile an authentic history of San Francisco's extraordinary past twenty-five years, I have maintained an amoralistic tone. Jane Addams explained the approach she took to listening to narratives of another misunderstood group, the visitors to her Hull House. "The Settlement House Movement," she argued, "does not lay so much stress on one set of virtues, but views the man in his moral aspects" (Franklin, 1986). Instead of diagnosing, she sought to listen, meeting guests where they were, not where she wanted them to be (Goldstein, 1990). This project was executed from a similar mode.

Germaine (1990) has argued that sharing stories heals. Many life story accounts, or "healing fictions" as Hillman (1983) describes them, are of surprisingly high literary value. In line with the tradition of Borges, in which any text is up for literary interpretation or juxtaposition, regardless of format, many therapists, Hillman included, have emphasized the use of the case history as fiction or literary narrative (see Phillips, 1994).

The recollections constituting this work come in the voices of people in hospital beds and living rooms sharing memories of friends and worlds long past. Through the oral history telling process, personal mythologies, passions, and longings are recovered; identities are embraced and reconstructed as whole entities; individual consciousnesses are resanctified (Cohler, 1982). In demonstrating the intagible resilience of the human life, they remind us of the force of the individual voice.

I have sought to allow those who have watched the plague from the very beginning to share their stories. In five years there may not be any more survivors from the epidemic's early years. Others must bear witness to the lost family members, the dementia, the young left as widows, the budget cuts, the women dead who were never diagnosed, the condescending doctors, the foot-dragging, the wasting syndrome, the weekly obits, the emotionally shell-shocked, those who died by themselves in hospital beds, those who have watched sixty or seventy friends die, those we loved who lost their minds to the tragedy and the humanity of AIDS.

The first generation of AIDS is over

Across the world, people have created a movement to fight AIDS. San Francisco's contribution to this fight grew out of the Gay Liberation Movement (Jones, 1995). The infrastructure and spirit of community activism Harvey Milk helped organize significantly contributed to the unique ethos with which the San Francisco Gay community was able to create an internationally renowned model of AIDS services, dubbed "The San Francisco Model" (see Shilts, 1987: 11–53; Fernandez, 1991). Federal AIDS relief monies would eventually be allocated to service strategies functioning along the guidelines of the San Francisco Model (see Hilts, 1990). By November 4, 1994, while most every other progressive in the land was mourning, San Franciscans cheered because they had played a key role in electing Tom Ammiano, the third openly gay member of the San Francisco Board of Supervisors. His election over a moderate Republican candidate insured the already progressive majority coalition on the Board would become even more liberal in the coming term (Stryker and Buskirk, 1996: 99). And eighteen years after Milk's death, the movement he led would come within one vote of passing comprehensive gay civil rights anti-discrimination legislation in a Republican-majority US Senate (Moss, 1997).

At a huge cost, Stonewall lurched forward. Kaposi's Sarcoma brought death, disease and queerness irretrievably out of the closet. Previously hushed whispers around ballooning health care costs turned to screams and all America benefited. The San Francisco AIDS story is a tale of how gay rights became human rights.

The interviews composing this history were taken from 1994 through 1995, fifteen years into the epidemic. The optimism of the Vancouver International AIDS Conference was still lifetimes away. The years 1994 and 1995 culminated in what looked like a frustrating dead end for AIDS activism and research. With the Concord Data recognizing AZT's "limited usefulness," a Democratic President in the White House, and reports that a second wave of infection had begun, HIV/AIDS entered a second generation with few solid answers ("The Second Wave," Gross, 1993). At the International AIDS Conference in Yokohama in 1994, Jonathan M. Mann, Harvard Professor of Epidemiology, acknowledged the need for rethinking: "It is now evident to all that while the first period, the first global AIDS strategy and all our work based upon it, was courageous, extremely important and necessary, it is also manifestly insufficient to bring the pandemic under control" (Pollack, 1994). I entered the interviews believing that PWAs, having had the most at stake, have a unique perspective with which to offer insights into the strengths and weaknesses of the First Generation of the interventions attempting to keep the epidemic's rampage in check.

"AIDS and the way we handled it can be seen as a model for a range of problems," activist Hank Wilson explained. AIDS fits into a mosaic of American poverty. Within the history of the AIDS pandemic, a cautionary tale on the complexities of tackling American social problems unfolds. We see the excitement and community vitality when volunteers lined up in force to serve their communities during the mid-1980s, only to watch these grass-roots organizations lose sight of their original goals and become bureaucratic monsters. Debilitating community infighting ensued. The AIDS fight has something to teach all those interested in addressing the array of American social problems.

Instead of re-verbalizing considerations of AIDS policy on a macro level, I documented a series of choices PWAs have made for their lives. Instead of a common historical thread weaving through the various interviews, I found that everyone chooses his or her own priorities. In a time when the conventional wisdom of the first generation of AIDS advocates has come into question, PWAs must choose for themselves how they best believe they can take on this disease. Life with HIV offers no absolutes, in the same way that the years after World War I presented few certainties for the survivors. Neither the government nor, until recently, the medical establishment has offered solid solutions. PWAs often know more about the disease or how their bodies are functioning than their doctors. Like the ever mutating nature of the virus itself, I found a range of strategies for battling both the disease and the industry surrounding it. Some interviewees chose to become activists. Others chose to look inward. Others challenged themselves to take care of those closest to them. Every person in whom the disease becomes active must live with choices about what to do with limited time. When every cough could be the beginning of a bad day, possibly a trip to the hospital, maybe a month-long stay or a taxi ride leading to the final destination of a hospital bed, the arena of choice becomes critical. These are personal accounts of choices made with information in constant flux, telling this fundamentally American story of the past seventeen years, as HIV slowly became another fixture and failure on the American historical, political landscape.

1988, bad news, and a trip back home

Raoul Thomas It's just, all the questions came up at once. Who do I tell? How do I tell them? What do I tell my family? How do I talk to lovers, all the people I have slept with? How far back? All of those questions came up really quickly. But that first day afterwards, I just remember, I couldn't deal with all those questions at once. Suddenly you feel like you're told that your life is going to be condensed to two years, too many major issues come up. Everything became urgent. You have to plan for your life and plan for your death at the same time. When you're in the middle of all that, you get these things from left field like, suddenly close friends begin to die, former roommates begin to die. My doctor died. One of my favorite professors in school died. All within a very short time.

Mom was incredibly supportive, I think I even told her that first week. That was my signal to tell people. I went back to Connecticut. I'm from a big family. There's thirteen of us altogether so there were a lot of people to tell, to sort of explain this to. Each one of them has their own families and they don't know what life was like during that time period Before. From the mid-'70s through the mid-'80s, it was everything that Armistead Maupin talked about in *Tales of the City* times a hundred. That was just a tiny glimpse into it. It was a supermarket of sex back then, everywhere. It was delicious. You couldn't not take a bite.

I always wondered how you could walk. There was no way to not be in on it and how could they not be in ecstasy. By the time I had arrived in the mid-'70s, it was just getting to its peak. It was like the fruit that was in season at that time. You took more than a bite, you just did, unless you were a celibate minister. Everybody was having sex with everybody. That was pretty much how it was then. Besides the bathhouses, there were even bisexual bathhouses back then, but there were also parties. People really did have orgies. The word was out that sex was good. Sex was OK. It wasn't so in the '50s and the '60s, but by the time the mid-'70s came around it was fun. Let's practice it.

When I first moved here, I was in North Beach. Polk Street was starting to happen. I remember Castro Street was totally different back then; I got off the bus at Castro and Market, "Wow, this was happening too."

Raoul began coming out to his family, in terms of both sexuality and health status, with a recollection of the story of his life, of the 1970s in San Francisco, when it was all new. So does this history.

Interviewee Biographical Notes

Art, *The Ghost Dance Continues*
Doomed to die in a hospice, he moved out weeks later . . . "All those 'what ifs' were sucking the life out of me." A Catholic priest, he called himself a "healing worker." He moved to San Francisco from New York in 1982. He died in 1994.

Hazel Betsey, *Hazel's Systems*
From Hartford to San Francisco to Seattle, back to Hartford to die, to San Francisco in 1995 to live again, from Jehovah's Witnesses to homelessness to a clean start. Today Hazel volunteers for WORLD.

Philip Blazer, *A Life within a Picture Frame*
A teacher, his Baptist minister father now delivers sermons to his congregation about the need for the Church to respond to AIDS. Moved to San Francisco. He died in 1994.

Robert Boulanget, *Tales of Two Lovers Gone*
Apartment manager from Quebec. Two of his lovers, Phillip and Tom, died of the plague. "My dying lover was in the bathtub and he was so skinny that the water was staying in the indentations in his collar bone." He moved to San Francisco in the mid-'70s.

G'dali Braverman, *Have a Happy AIDS!!!*
"AIDS activism is dangerously close to being on its deathbed." AIDS activist, formerly of ACT UP New York. Now with ACT UP Golden Gate. He moved to San Francisco in 1990.

John Cailleau, *Bodies as Billboards*
"I don't think ACT UP has done a good job distinguishing between their friends and their enemies." Born in Oakland. Former T-shirt designer and PR man. Participant in the '70s' liberation movement.

Ronnie Ashley (or Chaka), *The Clay We're Molded From*
Former cook, then Shanti Project Case Manager. Now he works at the
Native American AIDS Project. Moved to San Francisco after a childhood
on a reservation in Texas, then to Alabama, then Ithaca, then Texas and
finally to San Francisco in 1990. His life story is a case study in coping
skills and resilience.

Richard Chavez, *Unleashing the Keys to the Castle*
As he has watched AIDS grow exponentially he's observed: "The shadow
of our country is coming through." Former Shanti Activities Coordinator.
He moved to San Francisco from L.A.

Darnell Davis, *Adventures in Low Income Housing*
Grew up in Los Angeles before moving to San Francisco in the '80s.
Worked in design before the epidemic. Tells stories of the loss of his lover
and of institutional social control.

Per Eidspjeld, *Towards a New Way of Living*
A Norwegian immigrant, his philosophy, artwork, '64 Silver Mercedes
Convertible and all this man's life is a spectacle. He recounts tales of the
art world in San Francisco in the '70s.

Mike Fandel, *Beyond the Politics of AIDS*
Engineer. "I have no idea why the AIDS community hasn't gotten on the
health care bandwagon, why we aren't in Washington right now." Moved
to San Francisco in 1979. He died in 1995.

Paul Greenbaum, *Betrayal from the Left and the Right*
"Every group has its particular challenge. For my father it was WW I and
for myself it's a disease . . . but in the end everybody dies." Works at
Project Inform. Moved to San Francisco from Baltimore in 1974.

Peter Groubert, *A Room of Pieces of Many People's Lives*
"Maybe eight or ten of my contemporaries from the '70s are left. Now
when I see them we give each other big hugs because we know we are
the only ones left of a generation." Former MUNI bus driver. He moved
to San Francisco in 1968.

Cleve Jones, *Gay Rights Are Human Rights*
Former Harvey Milk aide, founded the San Francisco KS Foundation and
the Names Project. Moved to San Francisco from Phoenix in the early
'70s. Today he lives in Gernville and continues the work.

Cynora Jones, *Another Example of the Inhumanity of Man*
The only native San Franciscan I interviewed. Formerly a member of the
Black Panthers, later worked in a Fortune 500 company, mother and
widow to a husband lost to the epidemic.

Yvonne Knuckles, *On Coming Out to Yourself*
Lives with daughter and grandchildren in Oakland where she grew up.
Volunteers and is a member of the board of directors at WORLD. Does
frequent HIV outreach work.

Bob Lee, *Recollections of a Tragic Hero*
After a friend died: "I felt a rage take hold. I walked up to the nurse's
counter and screamed: 'GOD DAMN THIS FUCKING DISEASE!!!'"
Born in Alabama. Moved to San Francisco in 1974.

Nancy Lemoins, *I Will Not Go Quietly into That Long Dark Night*
Moved from Missouri to Seattle, then to San Francisco in the mid-'70s,
to Paris in 1980 and finally back to San Francisco, where she now lives.
Her art is frequently displayed at San Francisco galleries.

Hugo Manzo, *Towards a Language of AIDS*
"Why are we losing? Because all the agencies persist in pushing this idea
of safe sex. There is no such thing. Maybe safer but not safe."

Gabriel Martinez, *My Dwindling Circle*
Gabriel recalls learning about HIV in Mexico before moving to the United
States with his lover only to watch him die and a diminishing circle of
friends dwindle, ravaged by disease.

Marija Mrdjenovic, *Towards a Female Paradigm of AIDS*
"Last year I had two T-cells. Obviously there is something more to this
than T-cells. There are people with KS who have 700 T-cells and are nearly
dead." Moved from Missouri in 1979. An actress. She died in 1994.

David Pattent, *Link–South Africa*
Tells the story of a childhood in South Africa and his days on the sugar
daddy/international gay party circuit, coke, tricks, and, finally, a crash
into disease. Fifteen years later, he's moved back to help his nation face
the reality of HIV in South Africa.

Joel Posner, *Interview with the End*
Died three weeks after I last interviewed him. "Ben, since we last talked
my dementia has kicked in." He moved to San Francisco from Chicago.
Died in 1994.

Marcos Reyes, *Flattening Out*
Tested positive for HIV in Mexico within a week of a planned move to
the United States. Recalls the problem of moving from white collar to
blue collar work in a culture which assumed he was born to garden as
opposed to using his college psychology degree.

Jay Segal, *None of This Shit Makes Sense*
"The exciting part is that we are going to get a cancer cure from this, but
I don't think I am going to be around for it." Works for Project Inform
hot line. He moved to San Francisco from Chicago in the early '80s.

Brad Sherbert, *The First AIDS Funeral in New Orleans*
Recalls first hearing about AIDS in the southern United States. Tells the
story of going back to Arkansas to die but death never coming, so he
grabbed a bus and moved to San Francisco.

Rev. Mark Stanger, *Narcissus & Goldmund and HIV*
He found out he was HIV positive after spending a decade as a
Benedictine Monk. Associate priest at the Episcopalian Church of the
Advent.

Robin Tichane, *On Looking Into AIDS, Not At*
"My first friend to die of AIDS, he was hospitalized by March '82. He
looked terrible. By July he was dead. It was too bizarre." An artist. Moved
to San Francisco in mid-'70s.

Raoul Thomas, *Tales of a Continued Malignancy*
A disk jockey. Participated in Pro-Democracy in China in 1989. AIDS
Cure Research: "It's like the light at the end of the tunnel theory."

Dan Vojir, *Three Lives for Every One of the People from Back Home*
Author, book PR man. At the White Night Riots in 1979: "We saw Cops
throw boiling water at the bartender. They did it to the cries of Sieg Heil!"
Moved to San Francisco from Chicago in the '70s.

Hank Wilson, *The View from the Ambassador*
Manager of the Ambassador Hotel, a facility housing PWAs. Moved to
San Francisco from Sacramento and participated within the gay liberation
movement from the early '70s and continues today.

PART I

Before – The Groovy '70s

Vietnam was tearing the country apart in 1967. People yearned to get away from the East Coast Establishment. Bohemia lived in San Francisco. The Grateful Dead still played in the Haight/Ashbury; folks were still hitting the road westward to sip up some of the beatitude. The Black Panthers were setting up child care programs in Oakland. Cal. students were getting arrested in People's Park in Berkeley.

By 1968, however, the deaths at the Rolling Stones Concert in Altamont took some of the steam, some of the naiveté out of the hippie counter-culture. Speed, not acid or grass, became the drug of choice in the Haight/Ashbury. Paranoia took hold. The icons of the era, two Kennedys, MLK and Malcolm X were gone. The Nixon administration contributed to the downward disintegration of the Black Panther movement, most of the leadership of which found themselves in jail. As the '60s faded into history, people needed a breather.

Idealism faded, but not everywhere. A riot broke out after a police raid on a gay bar called the Stonewall Inn in Greenwich Village. As the "Me Generation" ate their papayas, a new movement grown out of the ashes of the '60s began to take hold in San Francisco. The Gay Liberation movement was much more grounded in the here and now of the '70s, in the possibility of changing a world that hated homosexuals. Instead of mourning the end of 1960s idealism, Gay Liberationists reveled in the opportunity of a new decade, a new chance to make America a friendly place to folks everywhere coming out as who they were.

We follow San Franciscans through their first days when they first got to the city, through the glory years of reveling in the freedom of the era. By the middle of the decade Harvey Milk was running for office and San Francisco elected the nation's first openly gay official, only to watch him get shot within a year of his election. The interviewees recall those heady days preceding the White Night Riots in reaction to the short sentences of Milk and Moscone's assassin, former policeman and Supervisor, Dan White. Cleve Jones takes us through the pre-riot tensions, his organizing, the burning police cars, the raid on the Elephant Walk and his calling to the Grand Jury. "The riots stood as a declaration," Cleve Jones observed. "We all live in San Francisco," placards read a continent away on Christopher Street in New York City the nights after the riot (Shilts, 1982). Only a year later, people in the Castro district began dying of a strange cancer.

ONE

Go West, Leaving the War Behind

Interviewees recall their visions of the world of the city as the '70s gay migration to San Francisco took steam.

Transferring to Travis Air Force Base

Peter Groubert One of my best buddies, he was in personnel, came up to me and he says, "Listen, we're almost ready to transfer out of here. Where do you want to go?" And I said, "Shit, I don't know. Where are you going?" He says, "Oh, well I'm going to San Francisco." I says, "Great, I'll go there too." So when it came time to cut orders he just put San Francisco on mine.

I arrived at night at the old San Francisco International Airport February 22nd, 1968. Got on a bus. Came into the city. It was a beautiful misty night, got off at the old downtown terminal at Jones and Eddy, right across from GLIDE Memorial, and then I walked over Nob Hill down to Chinatown and North Beach. And I remember walking up Powell Street in the mist and everything just sparkling. It truly was a wonderland with the cable cars coming out. And then I went into North Beach and was just dazzled by the old North Beach with all of the topless and stuff that was going on. It was just outrageous. Now I was in uniform, and I went into this bar called the Off Broadway. The star of the show was Evon Diandruss. She was billed as having two of San Francisco's three most prominent landmarks. She kind of crawled out on stage and her act was trying to stand up with these two huge tits attached to her body. It was truly hilarious (*Big laugh.*) And people were buying me drinks left and right. I was a soldier and the war in Vietnam was going whole hog then. They wanted to show that they cared for our boys. It was just a hoot. I really enjoyed it. After that I took a bus, 30 Stockton through the tunnel, walked back through the bus to the station, got on a bus back to the airport, slept there that night and then the next day got on the bus for Travis Air Force Base.

My first day there they put me in with these two guys. They asked me if I'd ever smoked dope. I said no. They said would you like to. I said yes.

And they proceeded to get me stoned my first full day in California. We were in the army on duty. It was the greatest experience listening to Jim Morrison singing "Light My Fire." The next weekend, we went into the Haight and I got to buy my first dope. And that started me on my medicinal career. That was also my first introduction into the Haight/Ashbury. It was right after the Summer of Love when it was still going strong. Walking down the street, every few feet there were people with hash and grass and acid, mescaline, cyclocybin, peyote, whatever you wanted – dirt cheap and the best of it, flower children everywhere. Everyone was brother this and brother that. People hadn't really gotten into panhandling yet. There were still lots of free agencies for people to get free everything, food, shelter. There were crash pads. So it wasn't a problem. It was really beautiful and a lot of fun and I immediately embraced the lifestyle.

I was in Berkeley for People's Park when we tore up the asphalt. We listened to K-San so we were up on what was happening around the University. We heard that the people wanted to use this land and turn it into a people's park and the University wanted to turn it into a parking lot. We wanted a park. They said that there was going to be a confrontation. We turned out in force to voice our opinion and the police showed up in force to voice theirs. I'm going to say that they started it. There were several confrontations, first it was the cops, then it was the National Guard. That day at People's Park, legally they were right. They had the papers to get everybody out of the property. But they started shoving, of course, because people weren't moving. Now, what they do is they do it peacefully. They handcuff you; they drag you away. Back then, we weren't doing peaceful demonstrations or at least not that day. They start pushing. They have horses. They run the horses into the crowd. They start using night sticks and it doesn't take long. A brick would come out of the crowd and scare a horse. The trooper would get real pissed and charge the crowd and start batting people on the head. Then more shit starts flying and it gets going.

When I go by there now, it's kind of distressing. The original reasons why we did it have been diluted so much and all those people are gone now. It's almost like a lost cause. It was a flash point. The riot doesn't need to continue. You've started the movement. So it doesn't really matter if Stonewall is there or not. It's the movement.

Finding a place

In September '72, after years in a Berkeley commune, I moved to the city because I had come out. The first gay bars I went to were I guess back in 1969 in the Tenderloin. Those were the only bars that I knew. There was the Alley Cat, the 181 Club, the Trap; they were all dives, mostly drag queens and there were go-go boys and real rough, rough people. There just weren't too many places to go. On Polk Street there were quieter restaurants for older men. And then the doorways at night time is where you'd find people standing around looking for other people to meet to stand in doorways and that was kind of weird.

Then I happened upon a bar right off of Lake Merrit in Oakland called Two Jacks. There were all gay men in there and I knew it and it was very strange. I was definitely the youngest person there. They told me that I would probably have a better time if I went over to this other bar in Berkeley called the White Horse 'cause they had a younger clientele. So I found the White Horse and it was a younger clientele but they were very collegiate and I was a hippie. It just wasn't my crowd. Somebody there told me about a new bar that had opened in the City and that I would fit in really well. It was called the Stud.

I remember getting the address and I remember driving over here, parking and walking in. Now this is the old Stud that used to be on Folsom between 11th and 12th. I remember pushing open the front door and all of a sudden here was a room full of people just like me. They were all long-hairs. There was something on the record player that I could identify with and they were gay. I had found Nirvana. It was wonderful. Shortly after that I heard of another bar called the Midnight Sun. It was in a really nice place right off Castro Street.

It was a quiet little neighborhood. There were some other gay bars right in the neighborhood but they were different. The Pendulum had a black clientele. There was a bar called the Mistake down on 18th just past Noe. The S in mistake was backwards and it was crooked a little, that was the mistake and it was a bar for older men. There was the Hombre, a leather bar, where the Detour is now. Those were the only bars in the neighborhood. So I would go to the Stud and the Midnight Sun. A bar called Toad Hall opened up supposedly for long-hairs where the Phoenix is now. They changed from bright lights and flashing psychedelia to much more toned down earthy kind of things with the mushrooms and gnomes. I got a job at Toad Hall as doorman.

Cleve Jones *Former Harvey Milk aide recalls moving to the city and meeting his old boss.* I went to high school in Phoenix. Actually, the first time I came here, I was traveling here with a group of Quakers. I had come to the Bay Area to attend the annual gathering of Quakers from the West Coast held out at Mirage. I was seventeen and that was when I had come out of the closet. There was a gay Quaker couple at that meeting and they were active with the Society for Individual Rights. So when I was seventeen sort of coincidentally, because the Quakers were grappling with the whole issue of gay rights, I met a number of the real pioneers in the movement and then I went back to Phoenix and joined the gay liberation group there. It was a very repressive dangerous situation and I was very anxious to move to San Francisco. The spring of '73 was when I hitchhiked up here. I don't remember the day I met Harvey [Milk], I just know I met him on the street on the corner of 18th and Castro. He flirted with me and I told him he wasn't my type. When he started running for office, I wasn't really into electoral politics. I was quite the little radical boy. I lived in a communal house in the Haight/Ashbury, worked as little as possible and went to all the clubs.

It was an incredibly exciting romantic time because it was brand new, so everything about gay people was brand new. I am only forty but I do remember the old days. I just barely experienced them but I remember that when I came out of the closet, there were only two gay bars in Phoenix. One was in the back alley and there were no windows or doors. It was just amazing to come here and other gay people were coming here from all over the country. There was just this electricity, this knowledge that we were all refugees from other places and we'd come here to build something that was new. I'm sure I romanticize it and idealize it, but I remember it as a very happy, remarkable time.

Nowadays, there is this whole emphasis on the sex part of it and the bathhouses and how we were all fucking our brains out. Certainly that was going on but there was an innocence to it that I have trouble explaining to people. There was a sweetness to it. Even the bathhouses were not the sordid and cold environments that I think most people think of them as. They were very social venues in which I would sit in the Jacuzzi for hours and see everybody you knew. There were many times I would go there and not even have sex but just gossip.

Dan Vojir I went to a Catholic College prep school in Illinois. Dominicans and Franciscans were adored because they were allowed to really slap you around. They were so totally into S & M, it was not funny. We could have

22

gone around in black leather jackets and black leather boots and they probably would have loved it. We used to swim naked, by the way. It was considered very manly, the Greek Spartan thing to do. By sophomore year, I actually had a group that called themselves "The Group" before Mary McCarthy's book came out, four guys who were also very intelligent, most of them a bit on the heavy side, no athletic prowess whatsoever. The odd thing is where the group is now; they used to ridicule me because I used to say I just wanted to get up from the ridicule of my parents. They would say, "Oh no, you are never going to do that because your parents are too protective and they are always going to be there." Breaking away was such a total break and their lives just went in the total opposite direction.

Years later, leaving home, revolt of the son ...

I was dumped by this guy, getting two hours a night of sleep, going out every single night, lost the job, and I just thought, I got a little bit of money. I told my folks I was transferred. I had a secretary at work draw up papers that said, "You've got a choice, you can go to either Montgomery or San Francisco." We did actually have offices there but I didn't have a job. My parents were like, You've got to go.

I had never seen the city before in my life at all when I came in '74. I bundled everything I had in the car, tricked my way through Salt Lake City, Reno, through Denver. When I got out here, it blew out of proportion. I was a kid in a candy store. I saw *The Advocate* was actually sold in the streets with other magazines and cable cars, and tourists. It was a brown paper bag in a wrapper type thing in Chicago.

I wound up at the YMCA for two weeks. Then I got familiar with every single bar in the city and I would end up sharing a house on Marina Blvd. Like I said, I had a little bit of money, like four or five thousand dollars. I was like, Oh God, I'll get a job someday. I don't care. This is wonderful. I got a car, relaxed and set to really enjoying it. My parents, like all parents, were calling every couple of weeks in the AM.

Robin Tichane The climate, the climate was just temperate and even. It doesn't get below 40 in the winter and above 80 in the summer. The gay scene was far advanced here as to what it was in NYC. I think the things that were turning me on at the time were the big philosophical questions: what do you want to do with your life and how can you make a lifetime's worth of hours and days meaningful, not just for yourself but for a lot of other people? I didn't come out until 1969 and I didn't do any drugs until the mid- to late '70s. Those factors came much later. It was just more of a hunch. It felt comfortable to ask who I want to associate with for a lifetime. Those were more essential questions.

Vietnam was going on and that was a real eye-opener. Basically 40 percent of the country was against the war and 40 percent was for the war and forever 20 percent of the country couldn't make up its mind. The pro-war folks were not only inventing Napalm and jellied gasoline to burn people's skin through, they thought this stuff through and invented a product, Agent Orange to defoliate entire jungles. The environmental movement was real big back then. It was so morally reprehensible that I just had to do everything I could to stop it. The United States and the things that were being done internationally in our name were appalling. There were lots of other people who thought that same way. I hung out with that group. It was a pretty thrilling time.

Paul Greenbaum I left behind a lot of prejudice and phobia to come to San Francisco. The last week in July '74, I came up here for a week and I was somewhat transfixed seeing Oz and the quaintness of the city, the Victorians. August 1st, I was coming out of the Cannery and saw the headline that the Supreme Court had ruled eight to one against Nixon on the Watergate Tapes. That's how I know exactly when it was. I was so happy. I said: "This is going to be interesting." It whetted my appetite.

I just plunged right in. Hot guys everywhere, the Castro Clone. I had my lumberjack shirt, it was the mustache. I still dress the same, jeans, these boots. Now I say I'm an older clone. My gay identity was emerging. I think everybody in the '70s did their black beauties, their what was then called MDA which is now called Ecstasy. We did all that stuff. From 5:30 when I got up until about 6:30, that was work, and then I would go out several nights a week, meeting a lot of people. All of these people have by now either died or moved away. We are older.

Peter Groubert It was right at the start of the influx into the Castro. I was right at square one. It was the place to be. I moved to 4064 18th Street. The very next day when I came out to get my car, it had been towed away because that was the day that they decided to make it a one-way street 'cause they were tearing up Market Street to put in Metro and BART (Bay Area Rapid Transit). They rerouted the traffic down my street. So I lost my car, but it was great to be in the neighborhood and watch it grow, wave after wave of people from different parts of the country, huge influxes. There was a whole group of people from Georgia, these girls wore outrageous platform shoes and lots of gold lamé, cowboys from Texas, farm boys from the Midwest, all coming together in the city. Everybody went hog wild. They found a place to be themselves after hearing all their lives that homosexuals were sick and the best thing for them to do is to commit suicide. All the ingrained things fly out the window when you see a group of people like you that aren't sick. All of a sudden having that freedom also gave everybody a green light to go ahead and have a lot of sex, which we did.

Free to be you and me

Dan Vojir Later on in '75, again, I was just floundering around, I applied to be a go-go dancer at the End Up. I was in the cage, two shows a week and got exactly twelve dollars a night. People would grab me when I got off so I got real paranoid. That wasn't what I wanted.

Robert Boulanget I was an announcer at the '76 Olympics. After it was over I came to San Francisco. Easy to not do much in San Francisco, you'd go in the bar in the afternoon and it was full of people. I met Phillip at one of those bars, Toad Hall. He was on angel dust. That was Thursday and I spent every day with him till Sunday when I was leaving. It was the Castro Street Fair. I had never seen anything like it, so many people on the street. That was different than it is now; I liked it better. It was smaller and quaint. We were there at the beginning. I guess it was more family; no wonder everybody slept with everybody.

Peter Groubert I went to an Easter Party up at 711 Corbit. They emptied furniture from all of the back rooms. A huge patio overlooked the entire city. They covered all the rooms in mattresses. There were candles. When we entered, there was a clothes check. There was a huge stack of little cans of Crisco. There were holders filled with rolled joints on all the tables around the apartment, cocaine, acid, and speed. And all of the hottest men in the city had been invited to this party. There were women. People having sex with everyone; women rolling around with the men. It was a true orgy. Everybody was high; everyone was happy. It didn't matter who you were doing what to or what was being done to you. You were there to just enjoy the feeling of it.

Every night was a madhouse. Every night at two o'clock. This was for several years, the end of '72, '73, '74, '75, '76, '77. Two o'clock, Castro Street basically closed. Traffic couldn't pass. Hundreds of people from the bars out in the street. The majority of the people didn't really want to have a lover relationship. It was kind of an ideal, but most everybody who wanted a lover, wanted an open relationship. People had open relationships and like most, they don't work. People were constantly dating other people so eventually you dated everybody and their lover. Everybody knew about everybody else. It was a small city, even though there were thousands of us. The baths went full force, pay a buck and get in for eight hours and just screw your brains out. It was quite amazing. There were just men everywhere.

Anything but the dating ritual

Dan Vojir I went from the super almost Archie Bunker structured environment to total breakout, total freedom. Tricking myself through everything but at the same time looking for a lover.

Peter Groubert The early, early '70s, people were just getting used to their freedom. Being sexual was part of that because all your life you couldn't touch another man. We always were faced with that, standing in line for the movies, or at the amusement park, there were always husbands, lovers and boyfriends and girlfriends hugging and kissing and we could never, ever do that. The only way homosexuals got to express any feeling was a quickie in a bookstore, an alley or a doorway. Everything was aimed at sex. That was the only thing, the only emotion that you were allowed. And even then that was against the law, sodomy. So all of a sudden there were thousands of us in a place where it was OK and the only thing we knew how to do was have sex. It was that or settle down like Ozzie and Harriet and we didn't want that. We didn't want to be straight but we didn't know what it meant to be gay or how to be gay. There was no book on it.

It went on. People just screwing and falling in love and having lovers and buying apartments and getting divorced just like the straight community. It's just that our sex was different and it evolved that way. We did have a lot more sex than straight people. We didn't want to have that big dance of meeting the girl, buying dinner, going to a movie, when they knew all they wanted was sex. Basically people just wanted to get it on and then if you get along, you become friends. Most people had sex and then became friends. When you go to a bar it's understood that you are there to meet somebody to have sex with. In the gay community it was just easier. People just cut through the bullshit.

TWO

Anita Bryant, O.J., T-Shirts and Milk

As the decade proceeded and the migration reached a critical mass, gay life began to extend out of the bars, the ghettos and villages to open participation within the greater society. The neighborhood grew and its citizens argued they deserved a voice in the city. Interviewees, several of whom had volunteered for his election campaign and the cause he stood for, recalled the unlikely ascendence of Harvey Milk to the San Francisco Board of Supervisors in 1977. "You gotta give 'em hope," Milk stumped. California State Senator Briggs launched a state-wide proposition called "The Briggs Initiative" to keep homosexuals out of teaching positions in California schools. The nation witnessed its first openly gay national official in action (Shilts, 1982). Interviewees recall the campaign led by Milk against a first glimpse of the Christian Fundamentalist Movement. The community galvanized in action around a man who would become the first of many martyrs.

The climate

Robin Tichane I was in New York in 1970 and it was a joke. Gay politics in NYC at the time of Stonewall was nothing, zero. I came out here and there were gay politicians. Harvey Milk was trying to run for Supervisor. Hongisto would go to gay drag balls. He would have his photo taken with a drag queen on either arm and it would make the paper. There was something called the Society for Individual Rights. All that happened in San Francisco in the '50s, twenty years ahead of the East Coast or anywhere else. So yeah, gay politics was already in place.

Vietnam had just finished the year before I came. 1975 was the end. There was a real relief nationwide. New York City was going into bankruptcy. Abe Beam had just been elected Mayor, he'd been controller. It turns out that all the bookkeeping he'd been previously responsible for had been screwed up. So in the gay world there were a lot of people who were wanting to leave New York. Economically, New York was not really taking off in the '70s and politically things were far superior out here, especially San Francisco – literally tens of thousands of gays and lesbians were moving out here.

Peter Groubert The political climate in the neighborhood changed a whole lot. Harvey and Scott moved into the neighborhood, I guess it was '73ish, and opened the Camera Shop on Castro up near 19th. There's a Skin Zone or a Body Shop there now. We, the gay community, started to get involved with politics in the city. We wanted a say in what was going on. We were still being harassed by the police.

Hank Wilson I moved from Sacramento to here. I didn't know there were gay bars in Sacramento. I discovered Polk Street, in the city, by chance and I started commuting for my sex life. After a while, I was commuting so much, I thought I'd better move. It's one thing to go on weekends, it's another to go in the middle of the week.

In the mid-'70s, homophobes would attack us right at 18th and Castro! Not on the outlying streets! The perception of us as a myth was that we were weak, gentle poets, with limp wrists who would run. Anyway, I ran into Howard Wallace. He was handing out a leaflet about police problems on Castro Street and I went to a meeting. That was the formation of BAGL, Bay Area Gay Liberation, in '74. And we turned that around. That's one of the important things I've done with my life.

I met Tom Ammiano [Tom Ammiano was elected onto the San Francisco Board of Supervisors in 1994] in BAGL. Both of us were teachers so we formed the Gay Teachers Association. We asked the school board of the San Francisco Unified School District for a non-discrimination policy in 1975. They put us on the agenda. We went to the crowded meeting and they wouldn't deal with the topic. After we left they voted seven to nil against us. They shafted us. So we brought the issue up at BAGL. The next meeting we went with our BAGL people and disrupted it *à la* ACT UP. We stood on desk tables, chairs; we hooted, we sweared, and said, "If you will put us on the agenda for the next meeting, we will stop disrupting this meeting." The point was, if you vote for or against us, that's one issue. But, you have a discussion of the problem. So they agreed and scheduled our topic for the agenda. That gave us two weeks to organize. We put signs in every bar and on every street pole in the Castro and Polk Street. If it was a gay bar, it knew about the school board meeting.

When we started to go political, our core group which was about thirty gay teachers, most of them freaked out because they weren't ready to go public. But Tom and I, being the arrogant/gifted teachers we were, we had the support of our faculties. They knew we were good teachers. So we pushed the issue. A lot of our traditional leaders told us that we were pushing the wrong issue and we were going to set back the gay movement because we were dealing with an issue of children. And it was ahead of our time. Harvey Milk was one of the few leaders who came to the school board. Other noted leaders like Jim Foster, they didn't come. The established leaders in the community deserted us and we won. Overnight a new generation of leaders was born.

Those of us who screamed at them at the board meeting lobbied the board members on the phone. I had told the board members that history was going to be made, that the choice was to be on the right or the wrong side of history. But we were going to press it if we needed to be arrested. We had a march permit for the following meeting so if we didn't win that night we were coming back. We wanted all the mythology about gays and kids to be put out on the table; we felt we could pass the test of the spotlight.

And we didn't know if the community would come 'cause we were a small group of teachers. When we got there that night it was really overwhelming. Three of us were willing to be arrested. Before the board meeting we had a rally scheduled. Hundreds of people showed up, people we didn't know from out of the woodwork. Lesbians came. Some even brought their kids and this was way back in 1975. Heterosexuals came. It was really exciting. I still remember the surprise. We marched from the ground floor to the auditorium for the board meeting. It was like hundreds of people walking up the stairwell. We carried the vote seven to nil. That was one of the first victories of gays and kids. We got employment protection before the college teachers did. Why? Because we stuck our necks out. That gave us a lot of impact.

Robin Tichane So, I was here in '76 and I'd see all my old friends from New York. People were flying back and forth. The Saint developed in New York making a permanent site out of large parties. These were people you'd see in the bathhouses. It was real community floating from New York to L.A. to San Francisco. Disco parties were starting to be put together. You could buy a share for $30. We had a community center down in Civic Center. It was a very happening, thrilling place. I was excited to be a part of such a creative community-based endeavor.

I had different friends who would handle different sub-specialties. I remember one man he was named Michael Maletta. Michael was a haircutter I knew from New York who came out almost at the exact same time as I did. He started a lot of the ideas behind the parties. John Cailleau was specifically into the concept of promotion. We would go into gay businessmen's associations. The message was, instead of it being in the margins, moving to the mainstream community.

John Cailleau We found ourselves much like a small town or a village. A lot of us were sort of the background action characters. When things were good they multiplied by virtue of the closeness of the communication. There were times at the Body Center which was the first gay gym in the city, when people would say, "Are you going to the party?" And everybody knew what you were talking about. There was only one party worth mentioning and that was one of the mega-parties that was produced with that energy from Michael Maletta and the two guys at Creative Conceptual Entertainment who are long long gone.

I remember going to one of the monster parties. As I walked in I noticed along the wall men just standing there, each one incredibly attractive with beautiful bodies. Every one had on one of the T-shirts that we had designed. It was as if I populated the gay community with art work, messages, and concepts that begin to become part of the culture. Where they come from, their origins, are even lost. Like that line, "So Many Men, So Little Time," was created by George Dewoody who is still alive, amazingly. George was never as sexually promiscuous as others like myself. He probably managed to avoid the dreaded virus.

Through the T-shirt business I was able to connect all my marketing skills through the gay community. We would kick up T-shirts which became reality-creating machines with messages like "I Want It All Now." So that there would be these fairly good looking men with fairly good looking bodies walking around with our billboards all over them. We attached a political message to our business. Personal life became a political statement. It was like having a printing press in the Middle Ages to have a T-shirt business in the '70s (Shepard, 1994A).

Peter Groubert The gay population changed the face of San Francisco. One of the first neighborhoods in the United States to be gentrified was the Castro. Gay men started moving in and fixing up the Victorians, painting them different colors. All of a sudden they went from those horrible old, broken down Victorians that they were tearing down by the thousands to those grand painted ladies. Property values started going up. People started coming into the neighborhood. It drew more and we wanted more of a say in what went on in the city.

John Cailleau Sylvester at the Symphony Hall! It was pretty outrageous seeing some black disco queen singing in the opera house. That was a time when for the first time all that you had been living under, self-imposed or socially imposed, was smashed. You were able to participate in the whole society, not just the gay bars.

I came to San Francisco to become a professional faggot. I say that because I was doing so much advocacy work that it was like another job. David Grisdine coined the phrase. He also created the Advocate Experience. These were self-realization seminars with a lot of mind control, eastern philosophy and how to put that into practical work. They were delivered in hotel ballrooms. You couldn't go to the bathroom when you wanted to. It was some deprivation, but mainly people didn't get a chance to reach for their nearest crutch, be it a cigarette, food or going to the bathroom. They had to hang out with and realize whatever feelings they were having. David did these seminars in the gay community and ended up bringing a bunch of us together. It led to a hard-core cadre of gay men and lesbians who would jump in and take responsibility under either political or community feeling.

The Briggs Initiative

Peter Groubert It took several tries to get district elections on the ballot. After a few times they were taken off. The Briggs Initiative, the Orange Juice thing, Anita Bryant, all of that happened at the same time. There were two communities: the committed political community and the weekend warriors. The weekend warriors were people who were young, gay, some professional making some fairly good money. They liked to dress well, eat well, party hard and they voted for what the clubs said was the best. Few people read any of the literature or followed up. The political people, like Harvey, Dennis Perone, and Rick Stokes, were out in the street. The people from the older, established organizations such as SIR, Society for Individual Rights, the Mattachine Society become the backbone, the money people. They knew the old names and had the connections. They got involved with all of the clubs to try to get the populace involved. For most everybody, it was surface.

John Cailleau Anita Bryant, beauty queen turned spokeswoman for Florida Orange Juice, like Russ Limbaugh today. She started a campaign in Dade county about homosexuals like today with the traditional values coalition and "special rights." Anita Bryant started making comparisons between the healthy he-men in the Orange Bowl Parade and all those mincing faggots in the San Francisco Parade. I thought, let's get some of these "Mincing Faggots" in T-shirts that say "Orange Bowl '77" so it looks like the whole Orange Bowl Parade has been subsumed into the '77 Gay Freedom Day Parade, which we did and those images went national.

Peter Groubert We boycotted Florida Orange Juice and it made quite an impact. It got everybody's attention and brought the community together. All of a sudden, our differences didn't matter as much. We were gay and they were attacking us just because we were gay, trying to take away what little rights that we had. It's basically taxation without representation. Those were the years that truly got the community together. It started in '76. Here we had a common enemy on whom to focus. Briggs didn't want us teaching in schools 'cause we were a bad influence. Anita Bryant didn't want us anywhere because we were a bad influence against God. She started all of this right-wing crap that we have to put up with now. It was during that time that the gay community mobilized politically and got district elections put on the board. We picked outrageously liberal candidates and a liberal mayor, George Moscone, over the hometown boy, John Molinari, who the rest of the city was backing. Those were the most political years, '76, '77, '78.

Hank Wilson We went to Miami and studied the Briggs Initiative, knowing that what was happening there would come back here. Then we came back and put up street displays of the homophobic ads. I would stand back and watch people watch the displays. Our people could not believe what was being said about us. That generated cash.

The ascendence of Harvey Milk

Robin Tichane Harvey Milk was just kind of an odd personality and he specifically hated the Gay Men's Business Group. I remember going in to visit him once and asking him to join. He was kind of huffy and "oh, who put you up to this?" He didn't have that "we're all kind of doing this ourselves." I don't have any ax to grind, but he was a crank. He wasn't into how he appeared. He was a sloppy dresser. He was a brilliant talker. He did have language down and really inspired you. But his camera store had just the worst window displays. Actually, he had no window displays. He would take boxes of his Kodak developers and he'd push them against his front window so when you walk down the street you would see the backs of the Kodak cardboard boxes (*laughing*) as his display. You knew that when you went in there you couldn't see outside but you knew that was the camera store. That was his sense of promotion. It wasn't real sophisticated. He had gotten the shaft a number of times and he didn't choose his political battles too well, so he made alliances and friendships that got him into trouble.

John Cailleau I didn't have a warm and close relationship with Harvey. The only time he and I ever interacted he bit my head off over something I had said in reference to Jim Foster, a much more mainline Democratic Party gay man who gave a civil rights speech at the 1972 Democratic Convention at three in the morning. Jim had a more respected position in the world. Harvey made some snappy comment that indicated a jealousy or resentment of Jim Foster and his activities.

Hank Wilson We got behind Harvey's campaign. We registered easily 10,000 people. We worked the street corners. We did it in a way that was out of the closet. It was inspiring to a new generation of people who had migrated to this city for a better life. And then we had an opportunity. Harvey was a vehicle and we got him elected.

Robin Tichane Harvey ran for an at-large post and he was always the sixth out of five, just an edge off. Finally the city went from at-large voting for supervisors to district. As soon as that happened, they went into the Castro and he was a landslide. So he went down there and did good things. He was involved with our Gay Pride Center and the parties. For one party, they were having difficulty renting one of the piers, he stepped in and arranged for an alternative pier just in the nick of time.

Cleve Jones Politically everything was new. So I met Harvey during that time and was charmed by him. I was a film major; he told me I had no talent but that I should be an organizer. I changed majors to Urban Studies, got an internship at his office, and did that until he was killed.

Peter Groubert He used to ask me for inside information on MUNI (a San Francisco public transportation provider). He says, "You tell me the good stuff on MUNI and I'll pass it on to the board. We'll get something done about it and make sure it runs right." He was just that open with people. He was a really great nice guy.

Winning

Hank Wilson Anyway, we came back here. Briggs was also beating the drum. He was also in Miami. They put the thing on the ballot. I took six months off of work to campaign full-time as an out teacher. We did the radio shows, every talk show we were invited to. The early polls showed that we were going to lose two to one. We didn't turn it around by ads or by raising money. We turned it around by having thousands of gays and lesbians get their bodies out on street corners.

I think that it was an incredible opportunity when Anita Bryant attacked us. The whole Orange Tuesday "Save Our Children" Campaign was an opportunity for us. For the first time, the word was out. Talk shows were talking about homosexuality. There were more articles written about homosexuals than in all the cumulative history up to that point. We studied them, we looked back at the periodicals. We know.

The suicide rate in this country for young people peaked in 1977 when Anita Bryant kicked off her campaign. According to the statistics and the chronology of when it leaped, it was a regular curve and it bleeped up when she started her campaign. People were talking about the issue for the first time and their kids were hearing about it. People were so ignorant because we didn't have anybody out there. We lost a lot of kids because of that and we saved a lot of kids, because all of a sudden we were a visible community for the first time.

Cleve Jones It wasn't easy. You had a huge population of people coming to the urban centers to come out. And you had the emergence and the creation of this community organization that had not been tested. The first real test was the Briggs Initiative and we were energized by the Anita Bryant Campaign. I was out here on the street blocking traffic on Orange Tuesday. I picked up on the Briggs Initiative a year before it qualified for the ballot. I had a conference at San Francisco State where we brought in gay students from twenty-something campuses and we started organizing. Harvey saw it as an incredible opportunity. We never thought we'd win, but we would use it as a way to get people to come out. It was an incredible rallying point. It was the first real outpouring of activism and we thought we would lose. It was so astonishing when we won. I think people were very much aware that we'd crossed this threshold, that we had created a state-wide structure, that we had raised significant money, we had mobilized considerable numbers of troops. We were hot and we knew it.

Hank Wilson Cleve and all his marches, the community, if they did something against us, we got in their face, we marched. The call would go out to the community. The signs would go up and hundreds and thousands of people would turn out. And we turned out because we cruised at those events and we still do. It was very, very exciting.

Cleve Jones The most memorable demos were the first ones, the angry marches, like after Orange Tuesday and the election defeats in Wichita, St. Paul and Eugene in the late '70s. I would gather people at Castro and Market, get whistles and all sorts of noise makers, and we would just go on rampages. We wouldn't break anything. We wouldn't hurt anything, but we would block all traffic and we would march all up and down the hills. (*Speaks with enthusiasm.*) I would take 'em down Market Street, to Van Ness, up Van Ness to California, up California, around Grace Cathedral, down Powell Street, through Union Square, and back up. Drove the cops out of their minds. And we would do it at midnight, marches with 20,000 people storming through the neighborhoods blowing whistles and banging drums, screaming, "Gay Rights Now!" We'd make a line then we'd turn right and when they thought we were going to go left, we'd go straight. That was fun and very dramatic. Terrified the police and it gave me such pleasure.

Martyrdom and a backlash

John Cailleau I was touched by the memorial service held in the opera house. Here you have the entire opera house filled with gay men and women and eulogies. The opera house was the cultural cathedral for the city and it dedicated that evening to the gay community honoring Harvey Milk. That was an awesome jump compared to the "don't talk about it, don't do it, pretend you're not there, don't touch yourself, every sperm is sacred," Catholic environment in which I had been brought up. We had taken over the Opera House for a memorial.

Peter Groubert I believe those were the most political years: '76, '77, '78. And then everything fell apart. First Jonestown and then Harvey and George getting shot. It just knocked so much out of the city as a whole and the gay community in particular. All of a sudden the city started infighting. I was a bus driver for MUNI. It was incredible, the things that I heard, people talking about "Poor Dan White being put in jail just for killing a faggot." Couldn't understand it, thought they had done the city a real good turn by getting rid of that Mayor and that "Fag Supervisor," just so cruel and heartless. They didn't see them as people.

Robin Tichane He was shot and the mayor was shot at the same time. It set back politics in this city ten years. Then only five years later AIDS arrived and set back the politics of gay men in the city for thirty years. Since Harvey was a target and Moscone was a target, it was a very effective pair of political assassinations. Policeman White knew what he was doing and set things back five years. Yet the gay parades continued. The Gay Pride Center was pulled down and to this day, fifteen years later, it hasn't been replaced. I'll say it was torn down in 1979 or '80. So, without that, there's no focus for all these little groups.

The morning of November 27, 1978, disgruntled former Supervisor Dan White shot Mayor George Moscone and Supervisor Harvey Milk in San Francisco City Hall. Mayor Moscone had made a decision not to reappoint former Supervisor White, who had stepped down from his post as Supervisor earlier in the year, only to ask the Mayor for his old job back a few days later. The night of the murders, 40,000 mourners walked from Castro Street to City Hall in silence. The candlelight procession stretched the entire mile plus the distance down Market Street from Castro to the Civic Center (Shilts, 1982: 260–92; Epstein, 1984; *The Sentinel*, 1978).

THREE

The White Night Riots

Former Supervisor and policeman Dan White was found guilty of involuntary manslaughter for the murders of sitting Mayor George Moscone and Supervisor Harvey Milk and sentenced to seven years and eight months with time off for good behavior. The night of the verdict demonstrators burnt twelve police cars before the police retaliated in the Castro. "The night of the riot, I will never forget any minute of it, ever," Cleve Jones recalled. San Franciscans remember it as the White Night Riots. (For further accounts of the White Night Riots see: Roberts, 1994; Weiss, 1984; Shilts, 1982: 324–48; Comeau, 1979; Petit, 1979A, B, C; Craiy 1979; Epstein, 1984; Lorch, 1979; S.F. Chronicle, 1979).

Cleve Jones To set it up, Harvey and George were murdered in late November of '78. I think that we'd had very high expectations because we'd won the Briggs Initiative and Harvey was in office and then he was taken from us. Now we have so many martyrs that people maybe lose track of the power of martyrdom, but though gay people certainly have a history of abuses directed against us, Harvey was really the first public martyr whose martyrdom was something that we had all participated in and shared in. Of course it was a terribly dramatic situation and people were very shocked and the community were very mobilized by it. But then the winter dragged on and on and on. During that winter there were two things that really increased the tension by quite a bit. One was Diane Feinstein's delay in appointing Harvey's successor. Diane had been elevated to mayor. Harvey had left a tape with the names of four, I believe four people who would have been deemed appropriate successors by him in case he was assassinated 'cause, you know, he always predicted he would be assassinated, the queen. So Diane just kept delaying and delaying and delaying on this appointment. We were all organized for Anne Kronenberg. At the same time the delay in the appointment was happening, the police started doing shit that they hadn't done in a long time.

All of a sudden there was this police presence in the bars. They were coming in and hassling people on Castro Street. I myself was asked for ID sitting on my stoop in front of my apartment building, and just weird, petty, bullshit harassment that we hadn't seen from the cops in several years. And then a group of police officers off duty invaded a lesbian bar off Geary street called Peg's Place (see Smith, 1979; Shilts, 1982: 306). They went in and beat up a number of women there including the owner, Linda Demarco. People were just really tense and really pissed off at the police. Also the trial was going on of Dan White. The general impression of the District Attorney, Joe Flavis, was that he was not pursuing the case aggressively. Others talked of the complexion of the jury ending up all white, mostly Catholic, all straight older people (see Petit, 1979A). There was not a black person on the jury or a gay person. So the stage was set.

About two weeks before the riots, which was May 21st, I was on Castro Street. It was a weekend in which the Milk Club leadership had gone for a retreat up here at the river and I didn't go. I was hanging out on Castro Street. There were these patrol specials, rent-a-cop type guys, and he was arresting somebody for putting up a flyer on a telephone pole. I was standing right there. I started yelling, "Why the hell can't you go and prevent crime or something? How many rapes and murders are going on and you are arresting this guy for putting up a poster?" A crowd began to gather to prevent the arrest. It was just amazing because it was a sunny Saturday afternoon on Castro Street and all the boys were out with their shirts off. This poor rent-a-pig just suddenly found himself surrounded by hundreds of pissed off fags who began throwing bottles and cans and cigarette butts. He had to call in reinforcements. Finally they had several cops. The police withdrew down 18th Street. We strolled in the street and people began cheering and laughing. Some people threw bottle rockets out their windows. So I knew then. He was going to get off and there was going to be a big riot and that Harvey would love it.

I was trying to be conscientious and I went to the police right after that incident. On Saturday, two weeks before the riot I went to see Captain Jeffries, who was the captain of Mission Station which includes the Castro. And I didn't want to go alone because I knew that the cops hated me already so I took some reporters from the local gay papers. I took somebody from the *BAR* and somebody from *The Sentinel*. I went in. I said that this had happened and that I had concerns about the potential for violence if Dan White was convicted of anything less than first degree murder. He was very condescending. He said, "Oh Cleve, you have your little marches, you've never had any violence in the past." I had organized about a half dozen late-night noisy, permitless actions. He almost patted me on the head. I remember pounding on his desk and saying, "You are not listening to me. There is going to be a riot and people could be killed and we need to come up with a plan." Finally, I got them to agree that if there was a demonstration when the verdict came out that I would assemble the people and would march them down Castro Street to City Hall then, but we would not have a rally, but rather I would keep people marching because that was always Harvey's strategy. When people were really pissed off the idea was to march them till they dropped. And so what looks to many people like a very reckless and chaotic spontaneous thing really was much more planned and orchestrated than people ever knew. We were very careful and always had a lot of monitors and communicated well with the police on what we were going to do. That was the plan. We would march down to City Hall then I would keep them marching.

But then, in the meantime, a coalition of radical leftists had come together. They were called, I think, Gays and Lesbians against the Death Penalty. Now the previous year during the Briggs Initiative, Proposition 6, which would have banned gay people from the schools, John Briggs, who sponsored that also had an initiative that increased or reinstated, I can't remember, a strengthening of the death penalty law. And so these leftists had organized around the idea that this would be a good political coalition of minority communities that were very concerned about unfair imposition of the death penalty. They were more left-wing than I was; these were people that really were into socialism and anti-imperialism and things that I was sympathetic to, but I was really focused on gay, gay, gay stuff. They decided that they would call for a rally regardless of what the verdict was – have a rally on the steps of City Hall to make these political connections that they wanted to make about the gay struggle and so forth of what we now call today people of color. They had already done that and I wasn't in touch with them.

When the verdict came down, I was sitting in my apartment on Castro Street. We were watching the news or getting ready to watch the news. I think it was about four o'clock. It came across the screen on the television: "Dan White Convicted, Details at Five." And my phone began ringing. I don't remember, I think they said what the verdict was. My first reaction was that I got violently sick to my stomach. I don't know what the blend of emotions was and part of it was just disgust. (*Voice changes.*) I just couldn't believe it, (*whispers*) how outrageous, such a slap. It was like someone spitting on Harvey's grave, spitting on all of us. It was just so clear what had happened. This all-American asshole cop, Irish Catholic from the old guard San Francisco. There's no proof of it, never will be; I believe and most people believe that Dan White was manipulated by the Police Officers Association. I don't think you

BEFORE — THE GROOVY '70s

could ever prove any kind of conspiracy or ever make any kind of real case for it but I don't care. I still think there was one and I think most people at the time believed that too. It was a *coup d'état*. He took out the head of a city government and the leading gay progressive ally. Mayor Moscone had forged the coalition that is now the progressive coalition in San Francisco. It was his novel idea to bring trade unionists and homosexuals together, feminists and environmentalists, Hispanics and blacks, an unusual idea then.

Dan Vojir But there was another interesting thing that happened. At that time Supervisors were only getting $9,500 a year. Being a Supervisor was considered being in a half-time job. Everybody knew this; the reason White wanted to resign at first was because he said he couldn't live on that. And then supposedly his family said that they would try to make do somehow and they wanted him to continue as Supervisor. The Mayor would not let him back (after he resigned). They considered him disruptive to the rest of the city council. His wife opened a concession on Pier 39, shortly after that, called Hot Potato, which was sort of a French fry-fast food place. That took $300,000 and to this day I think people are still wondering where did $300,000 come from when they said they couldn't make do with the $9,500 a year salary that he was getting. You draw your own conclusions from that.

Cleve Jones So I went into the bathroom and puked and the phone started ringing. Everybody came to my house because my apartment on Castro had been an organizing center for many of the demonstrations for the last couple of years. So they came over to my house. Someone came running up and said that there were news cameras on Castro Street and that they were looking for me. I went and found Don Martin and Phyllis Lyon. We arrived at the corner of Castro and 18th at about 5 or 5:30, still light out. The thing was that several months prior, I had decided to celebrate Harvey Milk's birthday, May 22nd, on Castro Street. I had permits from the police to close Castro Street, put up a stage and have this enormous party. I had booked Sylvester and other fabulous acts. People were really focused on me. The reporter said, "Well tomorrow is Harvey Milk's birthday and it would take permits to hold this party on Castro Street. Is that when the reaction will be?" and I said, "No, I think the reaction will be swift and it will be tonight."

As I was doing this I was focused on the reporter and answering the questions and looking at the camera and the rest of it. Then when the interview was done, which only was about three minutes, I looked around and the crowd had tripled. What had started as a knot of people standing around me and Don and Phyllis and this camera had tripled. It was now a couple of hundred people. One thing I will never forget was scanning the crowd and seeing someone whose face was so twisted with rage that I didn't even recognize him. It was Chris Perry who was the President of the Gay Democratic Club. Chris, himself, is a very mild-mannered fellow. I couldn't imagine that his face would look so different, so enraged. He had a sign; it said, "AVENGE HARVEY MILK."

Then I told my friends not to let anybody march down Market Street until I got back. I ran back up to my apartment to get my bullhorn. My apartment was packed. People were shoulder to shoulder. All the rooms, the kitchen, the back porch were just packed with people, everybody just white with anger, very, very strange. We got down to Castro Street and there were now about five thousand people. I'm not very good with crowd estimates but a large crowd was blocking traffic. People were honking their horns. But it was unlike anything I had ever seen before because in the past these gatherings, no matter how political the purpose was, it was always very gay, this odd blend of humor and sarcasm and camp that gay people employ, but this time (*laughs*) there were no smart remarks, no fancy dress. People were just fucking furious, a very, very different feeling. So we marched.

John Cailleau The day the Dan White verdict came out for his murder of Supervisor Harvey Milk and Mayor Moscone I had just gotten out of the gym or something and was on my way home at the MUNI station over at Castro and Market Street when I saw a group of people waving something, saying, "Let's go to city hall." They were going to do something about it. The march to City Hall is something that is not a secret but it is not widely talked about. I saw there was some potential not for some fun trouble but some dangerous trouble when I saw the kind of energy of the group coming down from 19th Street and Castro.

Cleve Jones There was still some light. And we marched on Market Street. All I remember really of this was to keep people from running, to try to slow it down. I figured that the death penalty coalition was already at City Hall and in fact they were and had already set up a sound system. So as the crown swarmed down Market Street I hopped on the back of a friend's motorcycle and went ahead of them down to City Hall. I met people from the Death Penalty Coalition and said, "Hi, have you got a sound system?" They said yes and they had a generator so they had an independent power source and they had put up the cables going up the stairs but they hadn't secured the front area. So as the marchers arrived, people immediately pressed up onto the stairs right up against the City Hall doors.

At this point the police became really alarmed and sent in a line of officers in riot gear up onto the stairs to try to come between the demonstrators and the building. At this point there still had been no violence, no rocks thrown, only shouting. The police, as they came up onto the stairs, knocked over the generator, knocked over the sound, not intentionally because in the rush and the chaos and the press of all these people. Actually, I think the generator had to be moved because it was going to fall or something. So the result of all this chaos was that there was no sound system and I really had the only bullhorn.

I was just so confused and angry myself. For the first time, I found myself taking this position that my emotions were taking me one way and my brain taking me the other way. I gave some lame remarks. I don't even remember what I said, something like, "Let's not be violent. Let's not be violent." I'm not a violent person but I felt violent. Then the bullhorn got passed around. Everybody gave basically the same line: We don't want to be violent; Dan White was violent; the police were violent. We're gay people; we don't want to be violent. And none of it was really working 'cause the crowd was just seething. And then finally Amber Hollibaugh, she's currently in New York City doing AIDS work, she's a fabulous glamour and dyke, filmmaker, a wonderful, wonderful woman, she got up. I don't remember anything she said except the one sentence. She said, "I think we oughta do this more often!" (*Laughs.*) By this time, I was no longer on the stairs. I had worked my way into the crowd and I was just watching in amazement. The crowd went wild.

Then the rocks started flying and the police retreated into the building. I was about maybe ten yards out into the street and I could see people I knew, people who I knew to be just the gentlest souls ripping that ornamental grillwork off the main front and jamming it through the front doors of City Hall. The police retreating back inside. One by one all of the windows were smashed and then I saw this burst of flames. There was one police car was parked right next to the City Hall front door. The other police cars were all lined up right on McAllister Street in front of the state building. There had been two dozen, at least, police cars lined up there. So then the first police car burned up by the front door of City Hall and the crowd went nuts, then that glow. It was animal, yelled in the crowd. That's when I started getting really confused, "Holy shit! What is going to happen?!" Then suddenly more breaking glass and you could see that people were getting into the building through basement windows.

At that point I realized that there was a possibility that the building would burn.

Hank Wilson I remember when the verdict came in, there was no question in my mind that history was going to be made the night of the verdict. I think when the first police car was burning that symbolically gays had fought back. We weren't going to take injustice. I remember when the first rock was thrown at the first window, it felt so good and then every time a window broke, it felt so good for your life accumulation of life trauma. We marched to City Hall and nobody said, "We're going to have a riot," but I think everybody knew. When I say everybody, I think most people knew what was going to happen. I remember we got there and I remember holding back friends that wanted to go into City Hall. This was after the windows were broken. One of my friends, Jerry, he had gone mad. He had gone over the edge. We were concerned that there were dozens of police in City Hall with billy clubs and we knew that if somebody got in there isolated they would just be creamed. So we held Jerry back. So then in the meantime, the people were throwing rocks and we broke a lot of windows. I still remember the first window and you could hear it and everybody cheered. I still remember that and then more windows were broken and everybody cheered. It was like a catharsis for our life oppression, just on the windows.

Cleve Jones Now it gets really confused because then the police began moving and maneuvering. It's very unclear what they were doing. I don't think they knew what they were doing either. There would be one hundred marching police officers in one direction. Then we'd see more over here. And then the crowd scattered because there was the first attack by the police. This line of cops came into the crowd. They imitated Roman Legion Triplicate, shields all up in a wall and they beat the shit out of us with their clubs, eh, eh, eh, eh, eh, eh, eh. (*Cleve demonstrates and makes paramilitary grunt noises.*) And then they came marching into the crowd. Well everybody saw them coming and turned around and ran and then the most amazing thing happened. A solid line of police officers advancing on this mob that is fleeing and I started chanting, "SLOW DOWN! SLOW DOWN! DON'T RUN! SLOW DOWN! SLOW," and people began to pick it up. We had all these people out there, all these marchers and once people saw what I was trying to do, everybody got it. The chant went on, "SLOW DOWN! SLOW DOWN!" and the mob slowly began to slow down. And then it changed, (*keeps rhythm*) "SLOW DOWN! DON'T RUN! SLOW DOWN! TURN AROUND! SLOW DOWN! TURN

BEFORE — THE GROOVY '70s

AROUND! SLOW DOWN! TURN AROUND! FIGHT BACK! TURN AROUND! FIGHT BACK! TURN AROUND! FIGHT." And the chant would change and we picked up and then finally the whole crowd just sort of stopped, turned and fell on the police and the police line had been stretched and we broke through them. Then we chased them back past the state building and then those police cars broke up in flames one after the other. It was so easy, you just kick in a window, light up a book of matches and toss it on the seat of the car and they went up in flames, one after the other, (*hits table*) explosions. Then the police start firing tear gas and by now it's dark.

Hank Wilson Then, we started going for the cars, when we got one police car burning. It was hundreds of people working together, not because they had met together. What happened was, the police would push us away and then we would throw rocks and the police would have to retreat. When the police retreated, people would run up towards the cars. And some people would break the windows of the cars with sticks. And other people and these were different people, would be bringing in the paper to push through the windows. Then, the police would come so it was like this battle of a wave back and forth. So, first the windows were broken in the cars. Then you'd have to retreat. And they would have to retreat. And then the papers would have to be put in the cars. And then you'd have to retreat again. Then, this next time when you got close to the cars, the people with the matches lit the paper that was already in the cars. It wasn't like you do it and it was boom, boom, boom. It was like this thing that kept going back and forth. I was watching for the police so we would tell people that were breaking the windows and pushing in the paper, when the police were coming because we didn't want anyone to get caught. And you have to watch from everywhere because you didn't know where the police were going to come and when they were going to charge.

But, it worked like that and I remember, we took over car by car. Pretty soon we realized we were working as a group. We understood the phenomena of waves. Like, you don't have to get in the car right now, but you're going to get it. So the next time we get near the car, have the paper ready, but the next time, have a crowbar or a club that will break a window. It was like we had met and orchestrated it but we never did. And, a lot of us never even knew each other but we worked together. And I remember people telling each other, there are people coming and then everyone would have to go back. Then, we'd get the rocks and throw them and they'd have to retreat. And then we got thirteen cars burning at once, it was just an incredibly powerful feeling.

It was also very scary, they beat us up and all that stuff but it was worth it. Image-wise, we knew this was being filmed and we wanted that image of us saying we don't have to just take this shit. We are going to fight back so then we did. And it was very scary too. I remember being totally petrified of police once we left the Civic Center area. They were hassling people and they were beating people up. I remember being isolated and losing all the people that I knew 'cause we were all going in different ways and then being totally terrified until I got back to the Castro. I came from around the Tenderloin; the police were going through the Tenderloin hassling people, basically driving people off the streets. I came back here and then went back there.

Cleve Jones My most vivid memory of the whole night, I think, except for the moment when the crowd froze in flight and turned, was when the tear gas started and I went into a reflecting pool to take off my shirt and my T-shirt and got my T-shirt wet so I could wipe off my face. I looked around and everywhere I could see there was fire and smoke, these silhouettes of people in the flames. I saw literal queens just throwing their bodies onto police officers. Then the crowd became more and more dispersed and the police formed one big line to disrupt everyone down to Civic Center Plaza. Groups of police officers on motorcycles were going up and down these streets just chasing down anybody and beating the shit out of anybody that was around.

I got pushed as far as east of McAllister, Powell Street, I ended up down at Powell and Market. Market Street was trashed down from Powell Street to Van Ness. And I ran into Bill Kraus, who was a wonderful man who died of AIDS early in the epidemic. He was Harry Britt's right-hand man. At one point we were at Market Street in front of the Bank of America. I saw him and we just started laughing at each other. (*Emotional laughing.*) It was so weird. I said, "Bill, have you ever broken a window?" And he said, "No, have you?" I said, "No. Not since I was a Cub Scout," and we were looking at this bank window. I said, "Well, do you wanna?" And he said, "God, just once in my life I'd like to throw a brick through a bank window." I said, "Go for it Bill. Go for it." He picked up this rock and throws it as hard as he could and it bounced off the window. So I'm falling down on the sidewalk laughing at him and I said, "You nelly thing, you can't even break a window. Let me show you how its done." So I pick up another rock and throw it as hard as I can at the window and it bounces off. So we're both just rolling around on the sidewalk just laughing in the flames and smoke and sirens all around us and we're just laughing at the fact that we're too nelly to break a window with a brick. And then this big butch bulldyke comes running around the corner, picks up one of those big garbage cans and threw the whole thing, smashing the window right in, and then reached in and set the curtains on fire. So we all looked at each other, "Shit, lets get out of here!" (*Laughs.*)

So I hitched a ride up with another motorcycle with this, I can't remember her name, she was this punk musician. She had spiky blond hair. I saw her going back with her bike and she drove me up to Castro Street. Castro Street was still pretty calm because a great many gay people when the verdict came out and the march started said, "Fuck that honey, I'm going to go have a drink. I don't want to deal with the cops. I don't want to deal with the radicals. I'm gonna go have a drink." So the bars on Castro Street were full of all these people that had been avoiding the problems. Plus there were now a whole bunch of people who had been down at the riot who were now coming back to the Castro. But it was a very festive sort of atmosphere.

Dan Vojir People say, Oh yeah sure, but I had this feeling that it was not going to stop here. So I ran over to Castro and I went right over to the Twin Peaks bar the first thing. I used to like the Twin Peaks. I said to a couple of people, "Do you know what's happening over in the Civic Center?" "No." No one in the Castro knew what was happening over in the Civic Center, no one. And I said, "There's stuff that's happening and police," and nobody would really listen. They were having a good time.

I had this feeling that it was going to move up and so I went to the Midnight Sun. In that day, Midnight Sun was right over in Castro Street and very significantly it had no windows and a steel door. I went in; I saw one friend and I said, "Something really bad is going to happen." I was really getting shaken by this time. He could see that and I think he knew the seriousness of the situation. Then it started happening. The police started coming down the street. We had heard some crashing because the Elephant Walk Bar wasn't too far away from us. That is when the police actually crashed through the front door of the Elephant Walk and then poured boiling water on the bartender and knocked the other one unconscious who actually wound up in a coma for about six months. They did it to cries of, "Sieg Heil!" and "Banzai!" by the way.

So we heard this crashing. Then they came. Cop cars were actually like a phalanx going down the street. You could see that. So then, the management in Midnight Sun closed the door. And said over the PA system, "Gentlemen, there is a disturbance outside. We don't want you to be involved. We don't want you to get hurt. We are locking the door." Well one poor guy was trying to get into the safety of the Midnight Sun from his motorcycle. He started screaming and I guess the cops were actually beating him, were on top of him by that time. We happened to open the door a wedge. He was bleeding and we got him through. The thing was, these steel doors, we weren't just in there. We were totally protected, basically, you know. But legally, when the cops said, you have to open up and kept on banging on the door, boom, boom, boom, the owners legally had to open up finally and they opened up. Everybody had to get out. All the men were taken out of Twin Peaks, out of the Phoenix, out of even up to the Pendulum.

Hank Wilson The police went into the Elephant Walk which was a gay bar at the corner of 18th and Castro and they just beat everybody in there. They broke all the furniture, all the mirrors. It was like non-discriminatory, they weren't targeting people that had hassled them. They just went in and did a catharsis brutality number. Then we got the people out of there. The cops finally left the area but it was a standoff for a while. The thing we did not want was to burn down the Castro. To our credit, we did show restraint and it wasn't deserved, we should have creamed the police right then. And we had the quantity of people to do it. But we had some intellectual love for our community and did want to burn it down. It could have happened very easily.

Cleve Jones Harry Britt and Bill Kraus confronted the police and tried to get them to leave. People were screaming at poor Harry, "Hey wow Harry, you've got the power now Harry. Can you do anything with it?" You know, he'd been on the job now for maybe a few weeks at most and people didn't know him very well. It was a terrible position for him and he told the police, "You don't belong," which was televised then. That was when I started getting really frightened.

At one point, I can't remember when in the evening it was but it was during the time of maximum chaos. My recollection was that the Elephant Walk was the first thing they did on Castro Street. I may be mistaken but the way I remember it was we were all milling around. I was up by my house which was up on 19th Street meeting with people figuring out what the hell we were going to do. And then the police charged into the Elephant Walk. We could hear the commotion down at 18th Street, ran down there and it was a mess. There was blood on the street and people were screaming. Then the first sweep of police came through and they just beat the shit out of everybody. I ran back up to my house. And I had a telephone tree. I knew people in at least every other building on those several blocks. I was on the phone and tried to get hold of people and we had people bring their fire extinguishers down to street level 'cause I was afraid the police were going to burn our neighborhood down. And I remember looking across the street and seeing men on their roofs across the street with rifles or shotguns. I don't know which and I couldn't tell if they were cops or gay people but I did see guns that night and that terrified me. And then the police started doing these sweeps up and down the street where they would just beat anybody up who they saw. We were dragging all the people on my block, the police would sweep down the street and then we would run down them and pick up these people who had gotten clubbed in the head. At one point, I think I had about a dozen people stretched out on the floor in my living room and kitchen. It was right on my kitchen floor. Some people had been clubbed by the police.

Dan Vojir They took everybody out of all the bars. They said, "You have to get out on the street" and herded us to the center of 18th and Castro Street. In effect, they blocked off the street but only on three sides. Their problem was that they had no idea how many guys were in these bars. Literally there were 1,000 guys that they had dragged down there and only fifty cops. Then it was the cops' turn to get scared. And the guys started shouting, "Go Home! Go Home! Go Home!" They had left an area where you could go in and out. The guys were just shouting at the police. And the police, basically in desperation, just dispersed because they knew they were outnumbered and that they couldn't go back and get more riot gear. It was a peaceful crowd just basically shouting. It was only around midnight or eleven o'clock.

I knew right away that it had united the community to a great degree. There was more of a sense of a community of belonging to something whether it was in mourning or in protest. We were definitely in agreement. Nobody was dissenting. When you're surrounded by police and you've got a thousand guys and you know that all the guys are in the same boat and we're all feeling the same with that. None of the guys were siding with the police. That was definite.

It's important to point out that the people in the Civic Center and the people that were in the Castro were not the same people. This was a peaceful community in the Castro that the cops just completely and utterly landed on like Stonewall. It had nothing to do with what was going on at the Civic Center. Hey, what the hell are you doing to us. They knew about the verdict. Of course, it was a shock but it was still a peaceful evening. Some of them knew about the verdict. I don't think all of them knew about the verdict yet. People were trying to have as best a time as they could and maybe a little bit of festering resentment. Today probably, something might start in the Castro. But this started at Civic Center. We had actually seen Feinstein looking from one of the upper rooms. People were saying she's cowering in terror there. The Mayor's office really was worried. They had uprooted a parking meter. How the hell do you do that? I don't know but they actually jumped right through the front doors of the Civic Center.

Cleve Jones And the next day was Harvey's birthday (*laughs*) and I had plans to close Castro Street. So Diane Feinstein's office, the Mayor called early the next morning. Of course, no one had slept. And it was an eight o'clock meeting in her office with all the great gay leaders, Jim Foster, all these respectable gay leaders, none of whom could stand me. They were commissioners and I was just the long-haired idiot kid. So we were all sitting in this meeting and Diane was about to call out the National Guard and she's talking to all of her commissioners and I'm just sitting in the back, listening and thinking, "These people don't know what the hell they're doing. (*Laughs.*) I'm the only one in this room that knows what the hell is going on. So finally one of the commissioners, I can't remember whether it was Jim Foster; I think it was Jim Foster who said, "Diane, you have to talk to Cleve." And it got kind of quiet. I didn't know it but *The Chronicle* was already out. I hadn't seen the paper yet but *The Chronicle* blamed me on the front page. They said the riot began after a crowd led by a Cleve Jones. I said, "Well, I think that if you bring in the National Guard that it will escalate" and she was going to cancel the birthday celebration and bring in the National Guard and put in martial law eventually and shut everything down. I said, "No, you do that and there'll be an escalation. What you should do is let me have a party honoring Harvey Milk and George Moscone." And I said, "I have 400 trained monitors," which was a bold-faced lie. I would deliver. The other gay leaders backed me up and said that I should be allowed to go ahead and do it which surprised me. Then I left and I got home.

Dan Vojir *The Chronicle* had a page that was one full photo with no text just saying, "Night of Terror," showing the cop cars burning. The story was on the inside. It was the first time that I ever saw a page photo on *The Chronicle*. That was very chilling. The jurors were interviewed and said,

"We didn't realize that it would cause this much commotion." Oh, for God sakes lady, the guy kills a Mayor and Supervisor. Whether he was gay or not that's still the Mayor and the Supervisor – he gets off with seven years. This was just absolutely, hideously, so way out of line. Everybody was incredulous. People were backing us up who weren't with the community. People all over the country were saying this is the most ridiculous thing we've heard in years.

John Cailleau Anyway, the night of the White Night Riot I was probably home watching TV. The next morning I pick up the papers and see the picture of the burning police cars. I went down to work where I had the T-shirt printing place and within the next day or so some guy comes in, sort of the Radical Fairy variety, selling a T-shirt that he put together the night before using the newspaper photograph and some quick homemade silk screening. We ended up remaking those screens for them and doing a top quality print job.

The verdict came out like on a Thursday, Friday evening there had been a Harvey Milk birthday party or anniversary, some Harvey Milk something. Sylvester was slated to perform. It was supposed to be a lighthearted thing. Nobody knew the verdict was going to come out when it did but because of the carry over from the night before it had the potential for lots of fistage and flares. I was determined because of the kind of business that I had that I had to do something to express my feelings about the Dan White verdict and ended up doing these T-shirts because I was in a T-shirt business by that time.

Cleve Jones I got back to Castro Street and I just got on the phone. I was very good in those days at the mechanics of organizing. One of the effective things that I had set up was this informal phone tree. It really began with just a list of fifty people and that I had. My roommate and I would call each of these fifty people. That would get the phone tree started. Then each of these fifty people had ten people that they would call who would each call ten people who were committed to this and who had used it before. It gave us the power, literally at a moment's notice, to turn out hundreds and sometimes thousands of people on the street. I got on that and got permission from the principal of Douglas School to use the auditorium there at that school up on the Collingwood playground. All day long we were training monitors, plus getting the stage set and the sound system and everything. All sorts of people were just buzzing about what was going on here and the radicals. I was holding meetings with my monitor people. I was also trying to get some communication going with the police. They were very paranoid because we knew that there were people on our side who wanted the violence to continue; we knew there were people on the cops' side who wanted the violence to continue. Many of us secretly and partially wanted the violence to continue but it couldn't, it had to stop.

John Cailleau   I did these shirts that said "PLEASE! No Violence" and went to where the monitors were training for the event and gave them all these T-shirts. The idea being that there would be all these bodies throughout the event which would say the same thing like a billboard, "Please! No Violence," over and over again. And we were all people who had worked together, trained together from the Advocate Experience and trusted each other enough for it to just be easy going. I took these shirts, put a pile in the middle of the room and let people grab them.

Cleve Jones   So anyway, I was sort of paranoid because I was sure that my phones were tapped. We were doing things like setting up secret medic stations and getting secret legal observers. In those days, not everybody had a video cam but we knew people who had video cameras. We were trying to set it up so the whole thing could be monitored. We wanted those people to be hidden away to take care of anybody that got hurt and we wanted to have the best lawyers there. We wanted to have a mechanism for getting bail money for anybody who got arrested. Everybody was going to my house and, finally, when I looked around the room and saw that I really did know and trust everybody in that room, I said, "Listen, we're all leaving here right now 'cause I don't think it's safe here and we can't use this phone. Just come with me now." I took them with me away to another friend's house. We were there ten minutes and there was a pounding on the door and the police came in and it was top brass. They said, "We want to know what you are doing." I said, "Well, what we're doing – we're going to have a rally and there'll be a lot of music and no moralizing." "Are you going to apologize for what happened?" "I don't think anybody's going to apologize." That'd been one of the things discussed in the Mayor's office – would the gay leaders apologize and they wouldn't, which I thought was remarkably ballsy of them.

So the police gave me a radio so I could talk to them. And they kept trying to ask all these kind of questions and making kind of threatening remarks about how many officers they had. I said, "Well, please just keep your officers out of sight. Deploy them around the parameter but don't let them be seen here." And at one point I had to call the Mayor's office back and say "Look, this isn't going to come off well unless you can keep

the cops out of the Castro. There should be no uniform police officers."
So there were thousands of police officers hidden nearby in alleys and
side streets but we kept them off. And then I remember running back
down to Castro Street 'cause it's show time, time to start. (*Whispers.*) I
came around the corner and saw solid people, just solid people. Many
people were wearing hard hats with sticks and clubs. (*Laughs.*) And I
thought . . . The stage was ready; the sound was ready. I hopped up on
stage and I had this radio that Captain Jeffries had given me. I checked
it and "Hello Cleve," this voice came on and said, "We just want you to
know, we're in a car in front of your apartment waiting for you and we'll
be there when this is over," which I took to be a direct threat. OK, then
I picked up the microphone and looked out at this sea of furious people.
I remember tapping the mike, waiting for the sound to come on, bump,
bump, and I took a deep breath and started talking.

John Cailleau We created an energy field within that gathering as well as
wearing the signs that kept the thing from getting out of hand.

Cleve Jones There was great music and speeches and humor and no
violence at all. It went on for many hours. When it was finally over a few
people had gotten drunk. That was the problem of staging a political action
on Castro because you had your militants that you could rely on and you
had the concerned liberals that you could rely on but you also had these
drunk queens in the bar, totally unpredictable.

At the end of the night, there were a few sort of drunk angry people
walking around and I had all my monitors. Whenever we saw anybody
that was trying to pick a fight, the police began to move in to do traffic
control and stuff like that and every now and then some drunk guy would
try to pick a fight and a little group of monitors would go around and
not confront the guy at all but stand around him and over and over we
would sing, "Happy Birthday, happy birthday dear Harvey, happy
birthday dear Harvey." We got through that night without a single act
of violence. When I got home there was a cruiser out in front of my
apartment and we went in. So that was the riot and the birthday party.

The Grand Jury

Then, you know, all hell broke loose and the Grand Jury was convened.
I can't remember how long it was after the riot. I've got it in a scrapbook.
I saved the subpoena. I'm in the shower one day and the phone rang and
this voice who I didn't recognize said, "Just wanted you to know that the

Grand Jury is coming after you." And I said, "When?" and they said, "Well, about any minute, get ready or leave." I was very scared of the Grand Jury because you know in the '60s and '70s, the Grand Juries had been used in very frightening ways to attack progressive political groups and individuals. Grand Jury, it was scary. About an hour after this anonymous phone call there was this knock on the door and that was the subpoena to come to the Grand Jury.

This is a wonderful story, 'cause I called up a number of radical attorneys, Matt Cole from the ACLU and a civil rights advocate friend and some other parties. In a Grand Jury you're not allowed to have counsel. No one can go into the Grand Jury with you. You have to do it alone. But at any time during the interrogation in front of the Grand Jury, you can request to consult with counsel. At that time I was a heavy smoker, so was Matt Cole. We both decided that every time they asked me a question, every question, no matter how mundane, every single question, I would stop; I would ask them to repeat it; I would write it down word for word; I would read it back to them, ask them if this was the question. Then I would respectfully request permission to consult with counsel before responding. So I went into court and they said, (*Cleve explains in monotone*) "What is your name?" I said, "Could you repeat the question?" "What is your name?" I wrote it down (*looks down, mimics writing on a pad, mumbles to himself*) "What is your name?" (*Looks up and asks*) "Is the question: 'What is my name?' I respectfully request permission to consult with counsel before responding." I go on up, out the hall, step outside, have a cigarette, go back in, sit down, "Cleve Jones." "What is your address?" "Could you repeat the question please?" "What is your address?" I write it down (*looks down, mimics writing on a pad again, and mumbles to himself*) "What is your address?" (*Asks court*) "Is the question: 'What is my address?'" "Yes." "I respectfully request to consult with counsel before responding." Go outside, smoke a cigarette, come back in, "521 Castro Street," or whatever my address was at the time. So this went on, it took them like four hours to get my name, address, occupation and school. It just went on and on and on.

The Foreman finally threatened me with contempt of court. He said that I was required by the law to answer and I was required by the law to keep everything I was asked and everything I answered a secret. So then I went out and talked with my attorney for some time and when I came back in I told them: "I intend to answer all of the questions that you ask me and I intend to answer them truthfully but it is also my intention to publish the questions that you ask and the answers that I have given." Then they went into an uproar. They said, "You can't do that. You can't do that." I said, "I intend to." Finally, they decided they would proceed and they said, "Please describe for us how you proceeded from Castro Street to City Hall." I went out and smoked a couple of cigarettes, came back in and said, "On foot." (*Laughs.*) And then half the jury cracked up and they were laughing. So they dismissed me and I was never indicted. There were charges pressed against some of the people who were arrested that night but there was no effort to prove any conspiracy. I think it was partly because the following weekend it was the Gay Pride Parade and it was just to everybody's interest not to see this go any farther.

So Sunday morning Gay Pride I was marching with the Harvey Milk Gay and Lesbian Democratic Club down Market Street. I hate to admit it but I had bodyguards because I had received a lot of threats. So we're just walking down the street and all of a sudden this sort of odd looking, very straight looking middle-aged man in a suit came out of the crowd onto the street in front of our contingent and started pointing at me, "You're Cleve Jones; You're Cleve Jones." And then the little group of bodyguards came all around me and we all went, great, he's carrying a gun or whatever is going to happen from him. But then he said, "I was on the Grand Jury! You were fabulous, girl!" (*Laughs hard.*) And that was it.

Dan Vojir   After that whole thing there was still a sense of community and a bit of moral outrage and everything else. The Castro Street Fair got even more raucous and riotous.

Peter Groubert   After Harvey died, the only things that brought the community together again were the Candlelight Marches and each year less people went to those. It kind of went back to the old ways, sex. More sex clubs opened. People just wanted to feel good. They saw politics as a lost cause. They left that to the Democratic Clubs. Trocadero was in full swing. '79, '80, I guess it was, Dreamland. MDA was the drug of choice. Sex was the happening thing. I have my diaries from back then and just reading them I get tired. The things I did were the things that most of the people did in '79, '80, '81 and even into '82.

Cleve Jones   I remember feeling exhilarated by it, frightened and uncertain how I was to behave but really exhilarated, and it was so amazing to watch those police cars explode one after another on McAllister Street and then we knew everything really was different; everything really was changed.

I think we did not clearly predict what the future would bring but we knew it would be different from what we had experienced before. And then there was really only a year or two. And I remember 1980; the Gay Pride Celebration had a Ferris wheel at the Civic Center. I was on that Ferris wheel with Anne Kronenberg and we talked about that and how we had survived Harvey's death and all of us who were around Harvey had been elevated by his death. We became prominent people and successful. We had accomplished an enormous amount in a very short time and then it all was changed again.

John Cailleau *During our interview, John frequently referred to one party he vividly remembers from the late '70s, one that he saw set the tone for the next decade.* The first T-shirt to start the whole thing was for a party called "Madness Takes Its Toll." *He handed me an old party invitation reading:* "The master's having one of his private affairs and you are invited to a private showing of the Rocky Horror Picture Show . . . Your ticket to the Rocky Horror Picture Show." That was from August 18, 1978. People showed up in costumes from the movie.

When we did that T-shirt especially, and I tend to believe that T-shirts have a way of creating their own reality, what madness was it that this T-shirt was really in reference to? Was it my own personal behavior and what kind of toll would it take? At that time, nobody had heard about AIDS. But I was wondering. Had my extraordinary self-indulgence and freedom in certain years or my years of dealing with hepatitis, were they going to lead to some dire result, some form of madness that I had engaged in, or were we talking about a larger cultural and societal situation, some kind of madness. And now in retrospect which is extraordinarily clear, you can see that was true, that the madness of the '70s, the Let's play, Let's party, Let's have sex did in fact lead to a consequence. So madness did take its toll. It was just a line from the *Rocky Horror Picture Show*. It was a free form of madness born out of a genuine spontaneity. It could be both divine madness and debauchery but even divine madness takes its toll (Shepard, 1994A).

PART II

The Early Years

FOUR

First Hearing

Within a year of the riots, men from the neighborhood were getting sick from strange cancer. Whispers, misinformation and omens of death dominated the discourse about the affliction. "My mother put a copy of an article about GRID in a magazine of mine. I thought she was crazy. Early on, we believed it was something that would only hit leather men, then we thought it only hit men in San Francisco and New York, then it hit my lover. That's how we learned about the disease," one long-term survivor remarked. Interviewees recall the days as HIV fatefully first crossed the paths of their lives. The die was cast.

First hearing

Robin Tichane   There were a couple of odd incidents of people's deaths maybe out there. Maybe one in '79, one in '80 but they were attributed to OD'ing on drugs and people dying shortly afterwards. It was hard to sort out, it seemed logical. I would have no way of going back and getting their names but by about '81, there were a couple of odd deaths. It was more than just one in a year, that I'd even heard of . . .

Peter Groubert   I first heard about this strange affliction that affected homosexuals by reading the newspaper on that April day in 1981 when it first came out in the *New York Times*. *The Chronicle* picked it up off of the AP and then they printed it in our paper. They talked about this cluster of homosexuals that came down with this strange disease and it kind of said that they weren't sure how it was spread. The article said that they didn't think that it was sexually transmitted, but they were not sure. It definitely caught my attention.

Cleve Jones   After Harvey was killed I got hired by the Speaker to the Assembly to work as a consultant in the legislature. It was a political appointment. I was the first openly gay staff person hired in legislature. But I was assigned to be the liaison from the Democratic Caucus to the health committee. I began receiving the CDC publications, including the *MMWR*, the *Mortality and Morbidity Weekly Report*, so I remember the first report. I remember being puzzled, alarmed. I saved it. Shortly after that there was a wire service report of what the *MMWR* had said, and I clipped that and put it on my bulletin board. I thought it was poppers. I couldn't think of anything else we did that straight people didn't do. Even the specific sex acts were the same.

Hank Wilson I heard on UPI, it was like a paragraph or two, a very short report from the Centers for Disease Control that there was a new phenomenon of people dying of an unusual pneumonia, and they happen to be homosexual. As soon as I heard that report, I went to the medical library at UC Parnassus, I mean, the same day. I figured that the system would not take care of us. There was no reason to think that the institutions would do what they needed to do. So, in 1981 I started doing research. I formed the community to monitor poppers. We were real concerned that poppers could be a cause of AIDS or a co-factor. We used the word co-factor right at the beginning.

I was a friend of Bobbi Campbell's before the epidemic. I found out that Bobbi had AIDS at what I think was the first meeting of the community about AIDS. Dr. Marcus Conant was also a featured speaker. Bobbi pulled me out of the room and told me he wanted me to know before the meeting that he was the person that had AIDS. Nobody knew anybody who had AIDS then. So he surfaced as a person with AIDS, publicly. Then, I think the next day, he came over to my house and showed me the lesions on his feet which was certainly interesting. At that time we didn't know too much and we were all paranoided out.

Vague memories and a first hospitalization

Jay Segal I met my first lover in Chicago where, I believe, I also became infected, to the best of my knowledge on Good Saturday, after Good Friday, in 1981. I was at a weekend party where we rented a suite of rooms filled with twelve naked boys. We had a crock of coke, a lot of needles, a lot of mirrors. We did everything including all over each other. I had my own needles. Dull needles hurt. There were two rules in our drugged, fucking, play group: everybody has to know CPR (cardiopulmonary resuscitation) and everybody hits themselves up. Those were our safe rules back in 1981.

September 20th the same year, I was in the St. Joseph's Hospital for some weird disease. Neurologists flew in from around the world. It was neurological. I was slurring my speech. I couldn't walk, I was bedridden, no bladder control whatsoever, out of it, down completely. Scared, panicked, no idea what's going on. They poked, probed, looked and they go, "We don't know what you have." I go, "That won't do. You poke and probe some more." They still didn't find anything they knew. They go, "It seems like you have multiple sclerosis but you don't fit the tests. You don't have multiple sclerosis but it looks like it." I had all the MS symptoms. Last year at the Berlin AIDS Conference, a French doctor named a neurological manifestation that usually occurs in sero-conversion. That disease was multiple sclerosis as in encephalopathy. Cephalopathy means your brain swells. It was MS like in the way that it demyelinates the nerves just like MS. But this is MS that will probably be a virus and is caused by HIV. MS is a progressive disease and this is not, and eventually will heal. I have no signs whatsoever.

I am convinced those are the times I got infected but somebody in that room had to have had HIV before. It doesn't come from mid-air; it comes from people. Somebody in there had it, could've been me. I don't know. I'll never know. It doesn't matter anyways. Going by that date in 1981 and out of that entire room, there are only two people alive to this day. We were all young puppies. I think I was the oldest there.

Lost friends, a first AIDS funeral in New Orleans . . .

Brad Sherbert It was 1981 and I had a roommate who got sick while I was living with him. He was a bartender and I was too, but we worked different shifts. I stopped in just to see him 'cause I never saw him at home. He was a big guy. I hadn't seen him in a while and I could tell he had lost weight. I asked him, "How come you lost so much weight?" He said, "Oh, it's this new diet I'm on. It's really working, you know." He said, "I feel great." And it was just a short time after that he went into the hospital but I didn't know they'd called it PCP.

It wasn't long. He lost weight and it wasn't but maybe a couple of weeks. At first they said he'd be all right in about a week to ten days with the antibiotics. Well, the antibiotics they gave him were obviously for regular pneumonia not PCP and they didn't work. After he was in there two weeks, I started asking, "Well, you know, you said he'd be all right in a week to ten days so what's going on?" They said, "Well, the anti-biotics aren't working." A few more days after that went by and he wasn't getting better. I knew at that point that he was going to die.

Just days before he died I overheard the doctors talking to his mother, 'cause she was wanting to know how come he wasn't recovering. And the doctor said, "Because he has no immune system. We did a T-cell count and we couldn't find any T-cells," and explained that that meant that he had no immune system, that he had a strange, very rare type of pneumonia that seemed to be hitting gay people at the time, that he was the first case in the South. There were a couple of cases in New York, one in L.A. and a few in San Francisco. They weren't really sure what was causing this immune weakness in gay men. So they just called it a Gay Related Immune Deficiency because all they knew, at that point, was gay men were getting pneumonia and cancer.

His family had a private funeral and none of his friends, not even me, were allowed to go. We had a private memorial service just outside the French Quarter. He had worked at a gay bar on Bourbon Street. We walked from the funeral home to that bar where we were having a private celebration of life – cocktails, food and everything. You would never have thought anybody had died. The bar didn't charge us for the drinks. We were there for hours. I remember, we got some strange looks walking down Bourbon Street. We had to walk through a straight part of the French Quarter. People were looking at us like, Why are all these gay people all dressed up and walking down the street?

Robin Tichane In '82 Michael Maletta, the guy I talked about who put together those first gatherings of friends, he was like an impresario; He was my barber. In January of '82 he wasn't feeling so good. Gyms were real big in the '70s and he went a lot. He was basically a gorgeous hunk. He was hospitalized around Easter of '82. I went to visit him and he looked terrible. He got out of the hospital but he wouldn't make appointments for me to get my hair cut, so I switched. Like July, maybe August, he was dead. It was just too bizarre; it had grown from maybe Christmas to July. Michael goes to all the bathhouses I do.

John Cailleau Michael Maletta was the first person that I knew to die of AIDS. When I asked a friend where he was 'cause I wanted to go see him, he said, "You don't want to go see him." I guess at that time the wasting and the KS spots were so uncommon as to be horrifying. Now people just say, "Oh, he's got KS," but then it was more than we could handle 'cause we were immortal, never to have any infirmities. You didn't see people on Castro with canes, certainly not wheelchairs.

One of the first things I heard about AIDS was a disease called GRID; that stood for Gay Related Immune Deficiency. I think it was doctors in Los Angeles who began noticing, maybe it was KS, maybe it was pneumocystis amongst a number of patients. It didn't fit the traditional profile for KS. The first person I knew to die was Michael. My line at the time was, "Once again Michael has shown us the way." He was the one that had created all the parties. Officially Michael was a barber and had a shop on upper Market. He did short haircuts of men who wore Levis and T-shirts. He was responsible for creating some of the visual effects in the haircuts. I created the T-shirts. When he had you in his chair he could impart a lot of enlightenment and philosophy of creative activity, some of the same stuff that I mouth off today. He acted kind of as a spiritual leader, a guru in his role as barber.

Chance encounters/information

Hank Wilson I remember, I was on Castro Street and I was talking to Bobbi and saw Cleve. So I went out and pulled him in and told them that they should meet each other because Cleve was a leader and they connected. That helped Cleve get the AIDS Foundation started.

Cleve Jones At some point, I met Bobbi Campbell. I was introduced to him by Hank Wilson. I was just walking down the street and saw Hank in the Twin Peaks bar; he knocked on the window and told me to come in. Bobbi had started writing a column for *The Sentinel* called, "Gay Cancer Journal." He took his shoes and socks off in the bar and showed me the lesions on the bottom of his feet. He was a member of the Sisters of Perpetual Indulgence. His drag name was Sister Florence Nightingale. So we did up a big flyer that explained the little bit we knew. We suggested that people cut down on their drug and alcohol intake and said that it looks like it may well be sexually transmitted but it was terribly hard to give anything definitive. Everybody was terribly suspicious. There were the beginnings of all the conspiracy theories starting to float around, kind of great denial and paranoia. It's hard.

G'dali Braverman In 1981, it was still just a "hmm, that was weird, that's sort of weird," "huh, what do you think?" "I don't know, what do you think?" "It just sounds like something isolated." That sort of general response. By mid-1982 it was clearly different. People were starting to shake in their pants. It was clear that it was more than isolated incidents. You heard secondhand accounts of those afflicted. Someone you know who had tricked with someone was sick and you didn't even know what sick meant because it was still something peripheral.

Art I never have tested. I got diagnosed in '82 before there was a test. There was no HIV; there was no AIDS. It was, there is, something was wrong. Basically the picture that came across was that you will probably die soon.

Cleve Jones Then I got a call from Marcus Conant. Marcus knew of me as an activist although I wasn't an activist back then, but he also wanted access to Agnos, who at that time had considerable power in the legislature. We have dinner at the Zuni. There's something about Conant's delivery that I believed what he said. That night he told me that he thought that there was supposed to be a virus, sexually transmitted, similar to hepatitis. Further, he said that there was a potential for a long incubation period. I think in that first conversation he told me about some of the clusters. One was a house on Fire Island where my best friend had stayed and there was a house here in the neighborhood. I did not personally know the people, but I knew who they were. Then there was a cluster in L.A. Then Marcus, I think Marcus has always known how to manipulate me, but he said that he wanted me to meet one of his patients. He took me up to UC and there was a man named Simon Guzman and that just was terrifying. His body was covered with lesions and he was near death. I think that he died a few weeks later. There was a picture of him sitting by the bed from when he was healthy, and I love Latino men. He was just my type. I was quite shaken by that and I think I knew that night at the Zuni what was going to happen. Marcus's delivery was so matter of fact. He led me through the bits of evidence that there were. He was jumping to a lot of conclusions but he was basically right. I knew that night.

That night, I left the restaurant and I thought that I would be killed by it, that everybody I knew would be killed by it, that they would find a cure but that it would destroy our community and our movement before. I thought that everything was in jeopardy. It was not at all clear how gay people would respond. Would we stay together? We had political power because we all came to live here. Why was it that we lived here? Was it only for sex? If we couldn't have sex, would we still want to live together? Would we have a community? What about all these things that had been created in less than a decade? The churches, all the social institutions. Would they survive? Would we pull together or would we fall apart? I was very frightened.

Dan Vojir In '81, I moved in with my second lover, Jack. He had been a guinea pig in the Air Force for drugs. You talk about it, they tried it on him. He never knew three years of his life; they disappeared. As a result, Jack got to be difficult to live with and things fell apart. I couldn't sleep with him. He would wake screaming, "Don't kill me."

It was still very sexual times, like I said, 1980 to '81. That was when quote "gay disease" was coming out. After I moved out, Jack said, "Dan, I wanted to tell you this. I've had these little things on me and . . ." He broke down because he didn't have any insurance. He worked as a waiter at Zims. He says, "I befriended this guy. I asked him to look at me in the washroom." Jack completely started crying. He says, "When he saw me, he freaked." To this day, it sends chills when I think of the way he said it. Jack was a tough guy from Hell's Kitchen. His father had a contract put out on him when he found out he was gay. He says, "And if you tell anybody, I will kill you." We knew that something was happening at that time. Word was just beginning to surface.

He decided he was going to move back to New York. He moved into a Franciscan monastery where he died. By that time it was already November of '82; Jack was considered something like number 436. I called to wish him Merry Christmas and I was trying to get through. They kept saying, "He's not here, bla, bla, bla . . ." So finally I got Father So and So, referred by Brother So and So. He says, "Well, we have to tell you that Jack died of cancer." I said, "No he didn't. He died of AIDS."

Robin Tichane Then a second friend that spring of '82 had this bizarre mouth cancer. He went to a doctor I also played with. The doctor says, "What is, I'll say John, concerned about? He just has a little mouth something; I'll go in and cut it out." This was a cancer specialist. All of a sudden he started sinking at the same time as the Michael Maletta thing. He was dead before Thanksgiving. My doctor friend was stunned. He couldn't believe it. He said, "Why would a thirty-three-year-old person drop dead from such a little mouth cancer?" Actually I went to the service with the doctor. Afterwards we went to a nice dinner and he said, "You know Robin, this is just totally baffling and something strange is beginning to . . ." And we came up with a few names.

Maybe by Christmas time the authorities had come up with a name for it, GRID. We kind of started realizing, oh it's more than just San Francisco. It's New York and L.A. It's gay related. Within six months, the Bay Area physicians had come up with a list of guidelines.

Peter Groubert More information started coming out and I started putting things together. I figured, whatever this was, I had it because I did all of those things that the people in the newspaper articles did. I got around a lot. I had sex with a lot of different people. One of the reasons that I thought I had been infected was the year before I had the swollen lymph nodes. I went to the hospital and they did a biopsy and they were not sure what it was. But I did look back over my records and it looks like it was the HIV when you seroconvert, the flu, the aches, pains and stuff like that. I checked my records and those were there. Years later, I checked with the hepatitis study and I had my blood drawn in August of '80. That was negative. Then it was just a month later that I had this thing with the lymph nodes. We called the VA. They had kept the sample and they checked it and it was positive. So back then in '80 is when I was infected. That was fourteen years ago.

So, in the meantime, here I was. I was sure I had this disease, whatever it was, although there was no test and there wouldn't be for a few years yet. All of a sudden, people started to die from GRID. One of my boyfriend's lovers, his lover was the first person I knew to die directly from AIDS. John died in '83. But even then, we still didn't know that it was sexually transmitted. So people were still having sex like crazy and more and more people started to get sick and die. They died so fast back then 'cause nobody had any . . . they didn't know they were sick right up until the end, which is one of the sneaky things about HIV. It doesn't really let you know until later on. So people were just screwing back and forth, infecting and reinfecting like crazy.

Venereal bizarro

Robin Tichane They didn't come right out and say it, but it seemed pretty clear something venereal bizarro is going on. The national authorities didn't say nothing and people just kind of started developing their own theories. I knew a friend who thought it was blood. He thought it was when he went for an operation, don't get a blood transfusion. He was kind of seeing it from that angle. And the authorities were mum, nothing nationwide. They weren't saying a prayer, none of this. More and more folks started to check out. The Bay Area physicians had their list of "this maybe," but it was guesswork.

Brad Sherbert I think it was in the latter part of '82 that I read they had found the reason that these gay men were getting sick was because there was a virus that was obviously sexually transmittable. They had no cure or no treatment for it and the results were always terminal. At that point, they didn't figure anybody to last more than six months with AIDS. But they weren't calling it AIDS then. I think it was either the latter part of '83 or the early part of '84 when they started calling it AIDS.

Robert Boulanget (*Apartment manager.*) It seems like everybody has slept here. It's very near the Castro, in the middle of Market Street. They had gay managers so it got gay tenants and was wild at times.

Unit 605 is a studio up on the sixth floor with a view. There were all kinds of stories about the tenant. Nobody ever saw him. 605 was pictured in *Drummer*, a leather magazine. It was like a dungeon. It had frescos of fist fucking and girls and guys, some kind of mirror on the ceiling, platforms and slings. The windows were made of mirrors.

And then all of a sudden this guy died. Apparently he'd killed himself. Everything in his room was so greasy. It was not to be believed. I took it apart and painted it but the fresco never come out. I rented it to this lady who moved in. Three months in, she called crying and said, "Robert, I cannot live here. I do not know what is wrong with here but I cannot live here." I think she felt the vibes. She said, "There is something about this apartment. I don't know what but I cannot . . ."

The story back then was, "I won't have AIDS because I don't wear leather." That's what we thought at first because it seemed like it was only leather people that got it. But 1982, it was just when you started questioning yourself whether or not you?

Peter Groubert People were afraid of themselves. They were afraid of everyone else. Fear truly gripped the city. Of course, the government didn't make it any better. As the older gay people died off and cuckooed and moved away, younger people came in.

Philip Blazer I was in San Francisco a couple of days before I saw the first report about gay cancer on KRON TV, April '82. I was with the people I was staying with and we all laughed. We thought, "What now? Everything about being gay is going to give you cancer. What now?" That was the first time I heard anything. It just progressed really fast to knowing a lot about it. I thought it was something that would never affect me. You know, they were finding these cases in places like L.A., New York, San Francisco and I was from the South. There's just no way. At that point I hadn't been here long enough to be promiscuous. And they didn't know how it was transmitted so that wasn't really a concern.

David Pattent So, the options were that I either left the country, or else I'd go to jail, or alternatively go into the military, *David explained as his rationale for leaving South Africa in '79.* I spent about a year bumming around Europe, specifically in the Southern Mediterranean regions. Got pretty bored with all that, didn't know what I was going to do for the rest of my life, figured, "Well, I'll go to Australia." But on my way to Australia, I thought, "I want to see America." So I literally got off the plane in New York and spent the next five and a half, six months traveling, tricking my way across. In Vegas, I was introduced to the whole new world which was sugar daddies. Wherever I went I was picked up by limousine, dropped off, you know, sugar daddies giving me rings and jewelry and buying me pretty clothes, and all I had to do was suck some dick once in a while, which was, you know, that's the way it went back in 1980.

I found a German lover, Tom, and got married to him. We built a home in Las Vegas and bought a boat. It was really a real fruity lifestyle, moving in the Liberace set and Wayland Flowers and people like that, Paul Lynn, Diana Ross, Cher. We were moving in some pretty high circles back there. We all were big into coke back in those days. Coke was – we all carried vials. You came into the house, there was this crock of cocaine that you just helped yourself to, did a couple of lines and went about your business, so, very much a way of the lifestyle back then. Then I met a man who changed my whole life. January 1983, that's when I met Bill. He and his lover Michael came on a boat. We were on a weekend charter on Lake Mead. He and I and his lover Michael hit it off really well.

Michael was a little head coldy, you could hear him sniffling and stuff, but he was having a good time. We were drinking champagne and dipping strawberries into champagne and having a real nice day. There was nothing to indicate that he was going to be dead three weeks later. He had a cold. In fact he had been in bed for like three or four days with a cold. And yet he looked fine. Well, not necessarily. Michael went very quickly. He wasn't one of those people that drug the whole thing out. I mean he got sick and died within three weeks. It was real quick, as was the case in the early '80s. People just got sick and died. It was, actually they had it easy, they really did.

Robert Boulanget My whole life was Phillip, nine years. When the first talk of AIDS came out I definitely did worry about Phillip and I guess about myself. I had done things back in the old days back in '73 but when I was with Phillip I didn't do much. "Oh, he doesn't look sick," people would say. There would be something following me, something there. At first I didn't know what it was. But it was big. It was like a rock . . . 'cause it was heavy and it was a taste and it was a feeling and it was there. You could not get rid of it. It was always there. Later on I realized what it was; AIDS. I was just aware of it.

Robin Tichane That doctor and I stayed in touch. In fact, today he's one of my best friends. It snowballed. It would become the topic of conversation at all dinners like maybe what opera people might have talked about when they got serious about opera. A lot of it was just hearsay, it was anecdotal, "Well such and such a friend died." People would get sick and die six days later of pneumonia and there was such a range of deaths. Some people would get some form of a cancer and other people would linger and get real real skinny. I had one friend who died of Kaposi's in his mouth. It was the combinations of ways of dying. It didn't seem possible that one thing could be causing this range of deaths. That was a bit odd, could it be related? Are the pneumonia people related to the KS people? I don't remember; it was jumbled. There was no pattern. Some people die of CMVA which goes to your eyes and you go blind. There are like thirty different ways to die. Those with KS don't necessarily get pneumonia. Could it be two things going on at the same time?

Bob Lee Those first years of the disease, the conversations over dinner and at the bars were basically denial. You know, "So and so I know has got the Gay Cancer but he was a slut." It was that kind of a reaction, "He deserves it." It just reinforced what we had been told.

Michael's death and this gay plague thing

David Pattent We met on the 18th of February 1983 and on the 10th of March Michael died, the first person in Las Vegas to die from AIDS. Big scandal. Bill was in the military at a nearby Air Force base. Hit the newspapers; they mentioned everything but his name.

Bill, Michael and I had become close. We hadn't had sex, but there was definitely an energy between us. Michael died. There was just this energy between Bill and I that I knew that he really wanted to talk; no one was listening to what he had to say. He was really hurting, but everyone was like, It's unpleasant, let's not deal with it. We don't know anything about this. At that point he had already become somewhat of a pariah, people didn't want to be involved with him. A couple of days later, Bill and I stayed up talking for about three or four hours and eventually wound up having sex with my lover in the bedroom. Fully aware of what was going on. This was the early '80s where promiscuity was encouraged. And that night I fell in love with the man. There was just something, an energy about him that I wanted to be a part of. I reached out and his pain became part of what I was feeling. It was a weird experience and it's never happened since.

I'd read the newspapers. It was called the gay plague in those days. Not even GRID. He died from the gay plague. The headlines of the *Las Vegas Review Journal* from the 10th of March 1983 read: First Gay Plague Death. Michael Shortell. I had just started hearing about this gay plague thing? I was kind of comatose to the whole thing. But when I read Michael's story, I realized that I, too, had this disease. Because everything that they were talking about I had manifested back in Iowa in August of 1982. The night sweats, the fatigue, I had come down with what were like flu/mono-like symptoms. I was sick for about six weeks. I lost probably about thirty pounds from night sweats. I just generally had this really tired feeling and didn't have any energy. So when I read the article, and the symptoms that were supposed to be part of this gay plague, a little light went on inside me, like, uh-oh, I've got this, too. So, when Bill and I were sitting talking in the wee hours of the morning and we started having sex, his comment to me was, "You have to realize that I probably carry this disease." Not knowing anything about it, of course, as no one did in those days, I said to him, "From what I understand of this disease I, too, carry it." I told him what had happened to me six months earlier and we decided that it was OK for both of us to have sex, because if we were both infected, what difference did it make? There was no such thing as reinfection. There was none of that knowledge back then at all.

Cultural impacts – us and them

Robin Tichane Before AIDS, a lot of the straight world found it a little chic to have a few gay friends. It was trendy to do that in the late '70s, so there was some openness that was evolving. By the time Reagan took office in 1981 and AIDS started coming out, then suddenly it evolved to where "this isn't quite so trendy" to have gay friends.

Harvey Milk got assassinated; Moscone got assassinated and Carter got thrown out of office. Mayor Feinstein had always been sympathetic to a lot of the gay people in the city, but she's clearly more conservative than Moscone, and Reagan was clearly more conservative than Carter. I found socially that things were shifting and bathhouses were no longer acceptable. They were eventually closed. My business, for two or three different reasons, closed. One of them was that I was an out openly gay person who ran it and people weren't quite so comfortable with it as they had been in the '70s. I associate a lot of that shift with AIDS.

Politically, it was conservatism triumphant. Reagan was elected especially on an anti-tax thing and he put into effect nationwide what

California had done in '78. After Vietnam people were kind of catching their breath. Did we really do this to the country of Vietnam? Just trying to ignore it. By '81, people wanted to forget Vietnam. They wanted to feel good about themselves. They wanted more money to spend, more money in their own personal, private pockets. All of that played into the situation of no special favors for marginalized groups in the country, anti-welfare. That paralleled those first four years.

FIVE

The First Wave of AIDS Activism

Cleve Jones The first wave of AIDS activism started in the early '80s and it was characterized by the buddy programs. There was this whole outpouring of people whose friends and lovers were getting sick. And we created Shanti and the AIDS Foundation and all that. It's very interesting for gay liberationists because we who had toiled for so long in such small numbers were suddenly joined by a lot of people. It was a little bit like the Briggs Initiative all over again. There was all this new blood in the movement and all these new people who had no political perspective at all. Most of us who had been part of the gay liberation came out of the anti-war and the Black Power movements.

G'dali Braverman *G'dali, born in Tel Aviv, moved to New York in 1981 after graduating from Georgetown. He explained his approach to the first few years.* By mid-1982 I had gotten involved with Gay Men's Health Crisis when it was all of literally twenty people.

The year before, my brother and I had met a man doing some design work in our office and we got friendly. He was an older gay man. I ran into him in the Village in 1982 and everything was happening. He said, "Are you interested in giving some of your time to do volunteer work?" And I said, "For what?" He told me and I said, "Yeah, I am."

I was twenty-two years old. I always felt that community service on some level was important. I wasn't wholly out. I felt that there was a basic urgency here and I couldn't identify why. I did not feel that I was at risk because I neither led a promiscuous life nor had I used any drugs. And even though, in the early days, we didn't identify that those were the things that transmitted the virus, it seemed on one level that those would probably be connected to whatever was going on. I never went to Fire Island or to San Francisco. I hadn't been in a sexually active environment. It was just something that I felt in my gut was important. In a corny way maybe there was some higher power there.

.We used to set up a folding table around the city, usually Saturdays and Sundays. There were like six or seven of us. The little information that was available was printed up into brochures and we'd stand at the table with all the pamphlets and a bucket asking for donations at 77th and

Columbus or down at Sheridan Square. It was really interesting to start getting a feel for the dynamic and the response on a very interactive level of the community and of the city as a whole. Most gay men would pass by the table or would cross the street to avoid the table, sort of the way that you avoid the perfume salesperson at Bloomingdale's at the bottom of the escalator. So you'd find yourself just disgusted with the community. But women with babies with strollers would stop; younger heterosexuals seemed to be interested or accessible on some level that most gay men weren't. Literally you could spend entire Saturdays and Sundays with maybe only three or four gay men ever stopping to talk or donate money. Of course, as the incidence rose, more people knew someone who knew someone who knew someone, then more people knew someone who knew someone who knew someone. And then more people were dead.

I can remember we had a placard. It was handmade. Everything was really very primitive. We mounted it behind the table and on the top it said: "New York Cases" and then below it said: "US Cases" and I can remember when there were 300 or 400. I can remember when we hit 1000 in New York and we switched the numbers. It was '83 . . .

Cleve Jones (*The early AIDS Foundation Years*) It was so weird, the day we opened an office we had a phone put in and it was not listed. By the end of that first day that phone never stopped ringing. There was a line of people, it was upstairs, down the stairs onto the sidewalk. I would just go down on the street and look for people whose faces I knew from political organizing and I'd (*reaches over to hold my arm*) grab them and I'd say, "Would you please come upstairs and answer the phone for me please?" And we did it. We decided that we had to organize. We sort of had found a cause. There was not really a lot to do except try to be there for people. Our first efforts were in finding physicians who were not homophobic who would see these patients.

G'dali Braverman GMHC was extremely disorganized. It was extremely difficult to do the work we were committed to do. One of the guys in our group had in 1981 lost his lover. By 1983, people that I had worked or volunteered with had become sick. People who came up to the table would come with concerns regarding their friends or lovers.

"The doctors knew absolutely nothing"

Art At the time nobody knew very much so I thought, I am not going to listen to you. (*Laughs.*) Although the minute anybody thought they knew

72

anything, they insisted I listen. I went to San Francisco General when I was first diagnosed. There was a list of tests that we were expected to go through, a whole page and everyone said, "Your appointment is here, here, and here." Once I was with the doctor I said, "Let's look at this list." Only one or two of them would do me any good and some of them were dangerous and painful. Nobody questioned it. I know people who have had their lungs collapse from bronchoscopies that weren't necessary. Blood gas tests they were doing were a painful process. You have to open an artery. Anything not to have fear, to pretend you've got something in control.

Early on I set to looking at the alternative treatments. It was a wonderful proving ground. This was one area in which the doctors had to admit that they knew absolutely nothing and were having no success. So, where else to prove the holistic methods? I took a lot of time into exploring how the body deals with cancer, how it can deal with it naturally and how there are things that get in the way – stress and alcohol and drugs and treatments that you are given for it, even from spiritual lack. It turned out that illness is not an isolated thing as we would have it. Dealing with it involves a different movement of art.

Somewhere there is a virus that either comes along for the ride or is caused. I don't know which and I don't care. Early in this process, I sat down and wrote up a list of things that I was going to do if I was going to die and what I was going to do if I was going to live. I worked on that, meditating and really analyzed those two ways and found that the more that I thought about it, meditated on it, the more they became the same list, and that the illusion that they were two different lists represented a split in me and living in a place that wasn't now. All those "what ifs" were sucking the life out of me. Those lists just started to merge. What I was feeling at that point should have been just what I wanted to and should do. What was going to happen in another ten years all depended on what I was going to do right now. The future issue just lost all of its power.

Confusion and responses

Hank Wilson I worked on the first AIDS Candlelight March. It was the first time that we put the call out to the community to support people with AIDS and again we didn't know if people would come. The parade was totally controlled by people with AIDS. We put up signs everywhere and again, we saturated. I remember yelling at a guy that owned a gay bookstore because he wouldn't let us post a sign about the Candlelight March. I disrupted his store and he changed his mind.

I called Larry Kramer and Paul Popham and told him that we'd send posters for the march 'cause we wanted them to have one at the same time and we knew that GMHC was having an event at Madison Square Garden. If they announced the Candlelight March all they'd have to do is turn the lights out and light a candle. From the beginning we had marches on both coasts. I called both Larry and Paul but I didn't tell them, they were already feuding, to make sure it happened.

This march was incredible; thousands of people did come. I remember the meeting where we came up with the theme, talk about process: we had a meeting for everything. We talked about different things. "Fighting for Our Lives," as soon as anybody said it, everybody consensed on it. That was what it was going to be.

Robin Tichane It wasn't until '84 or even '85 that they identified an HIV virus. When they announced that they had identified HIV, it was pretty clear that they had identified it and had held off announcing it until they had a test for it as well. It will come out in twenty years that between '81 and '85 the authorities knew there was a venereal disease and a blood infection but they didn't want the country to go bonkers. They thought if they could not identify this blood product, that for four years all surgery in the United States, all blood transfusions would stop. People would have been hysterical, so they said nothing.

I think that, say, within six months of '81, they could have come out that it's a venereal disease, you don't have to prove it, so use more precautions and we're working on the blood supply issue. Everyone was guessing for four years. I think the bathhouses closed before '85, based on guesswork. It's pretty appalling. That allowed many avenues of transmission to happen which were totally preventable.

Hank Wilson Gary Walsh went to the Harvey Milk Gay Democratic Club. I remember he brought this thing up. We were trying to talk about how the community responds about AIDS and Carol Migden, of the State Assembly, adjourned the meeting right in the middle of the discussion. She was president at the time. I support Carol now. But historically, he took the issue, as a person with AIDS, asked for support to do a march and they adjourned the meeting rudely. I was there and I went to him and I said, "We can do this." We don't have to do it through this group, we'll just do it and we did it.

People were very frightened, traumatized. Early on that was clear. We also knew people were getting sick. It was very difficult to deal with and then, was it going to be a liability for the community and for the political agenda? You had people using it as a political weapon.

There was that controversy about the bathhouses. I went to all those Health Department meetings from the beginning. There were also people who were making charges that went to those meetings. Process-wise, they did not raise their voices. And then you would read about stuff in the paper and I would go like, "I was just at that meeting. That could have been raised at that meeting," and it wasn't. They were getting political mileage out of it. I'm talking about, What should we do and how should we do it? Should we tell the community? And what is the message? When do you do it? Who does it? There's no question that you tell the community. The question is, what is the context? What's the message? And how do you do it? Stylistically, there are different ways to go about that. AIDS became a political football. Some people used AIDS and I still feel a lot of anger about that.

Peter Groubert A big controversy about the baths that split the community quite a bit back then. One side wanted baths closed, the other didn't. It was a health issue. It was a political issue. It was a freedom issue. It became so many issues. It was all pretty ridiculous.

Robin Tichane I saw some statistics about rates of rectal gonorrhea in San Francisco. In 1979, there were 400 to 600 cases at the city clinic every single month, phenomenal rates! By 1980, public health people in San Francisco were seeing 100 cases of gay rectal gonorrhea. People were kind of getting the message. The rate was 500 down to 100 just on a hunch. By 1990, it's down to 20 to 25 a month, a 500 percent drop. By 1990, they had to close a lot of public clinics because there was no caseload. But nothing about HIV until '85. Those bastards ignored it or deliberately hid it. That'll come out, there's a real story there.

The stories we'd get from the government were maybe it's Crisco. Maybe it's poppers. They were just kind of absurd explanations. It was all kind of fuzzy what was going on. People thought, "Oh, if we're goody two shoes and use condoms for these six months then we're over the hump." No one had any idea that it would take over eleven years and that people who are dying today weren't infected just six months before their first illness. It might've been eleven years?! How can an infectious agent take eleven years, average, incubation? We were all thinking in old-fashioned terms that, oh, six months for tops. But as it got bigger and bigger, well maybe it's a year. Could it possibly be fourteen to eighteen months? The concept of eleven years average was not conceivable, whereas today it's a fact. Some people thought that if you got a glass of vitamin C that would prevent it. There was a kind of quack medicine going on as to how it's transmitted and how to deal with it. It was a strange period.

Hank Wilson In 1985 Mobilization Against AIDS picketed Barbara Boxer at one of her community meetings. We were angry because the Democratic controlled Congress wasn't doing what it might do. Everyone wants to blame the Republicans, OK. She about had a stroke. She wasn't homophobic but she also wasn't being responsive. We were asking for funding, resources. We got in their face. We had a mentality which is we think it is important right now for younger gays and lesbians, "Don't Rely on the System. Do What Needs to Be Done. Take Care of Yourself."

Cleve Jones The fear in that first couple of years until 1985 was just a roller coaster tale for me because my circle of friends was hit very early. I didn't know it at the time but I was already infected. I had lovers and boyfriends who had been sick so I assumed that I was infected. When I look back I am also really proud because nobody did a fucking thing except us. I've made a lot of mistakes in my life and done many things that I really regret, but I was one of the first people on the planet to understand that this was going to happen. I was one of the first people to act. I knew all the people who were among the first to respond. We were heroes. There are many things I would do differently now but I still think that we did a good job.

SIX

Test Results and Time Bombs

Robin Tichane Reagan and the Hollywood folks had the imagery down and they were able to manipulate broadcasts and print media very persuasively. They had lots of practice. It was overwhelming to see all of those promotional things be put to effective use at the national level. About the time they had given a name for the HIV virus, they came out with a test. Those were almost identical events.

Jay Segal I was in the trial for the test in 1984. You still remember the counseling, walking in that room and them telling you the results. There are certain things in your life you always remember. If you're old enough, you remember when Kennedy got shot or when the Wall fell. I can even remember the guy who told me I was positive. I wasn't too shocked. I figured as much since I had already lost a boyfriend.

Time bombs, part one

David Pattent The next day, I went to my doctor's. I would like to mention his name but I'm not going to because he is very big in the HIV movement. He's written a book. Went in and I say to him, "You know, I think that I've been exposed to this virus. There is something going on in my body." My lymph nodes were all real puffy. So he did, what they knew in those days, a T-cell count, which took three or four days to get back because they had to literally hand count the T-cells. So, he called me back into his office and he said, "Looking at the way your immune function is right now, you probably have about six months to a year to live, probably closer to six months." The advice he gave me was two sentences: "Get your affairs in order and please do not come back. Because if anyone finds out, I will lose all my patients." I went numb. And it was just this, Okay, so I'm dying, now what do I do? Literally, I went out that week and arranged my funeral and got my affairs in order.

My immune function at that point, I think my T-cells were like at 362. So, I was already immune compromised. And of course there was nothing, no medications. So, Oh God, it's such a long time ago. I went home and told Tom. In the meantime, Bill had told his Base Commander that he suspected that he was carrying this disease. Everyone knew that Bill was gay, but it wasn't a spoken about thing because everyone respected him so much. They started running batteries of tests on him and immediately knew that his immune system was compromised. There were a number of things that had gone wrong. We didn't know it, but the Office of Special Investigation had already started investigating him for homosexual behavior. But they couldn't prove anything so they closed the file. When he came forward, the file reopened itself.

Ronnie Ashley   I started hearing about the "Gay Plague," in late 1980, '81, '82. I was in San Antonio at the time. In 1983, I had gotten real sick, what I had assumed was a cold got worse and I ended up flat on my back. They ran all these tests. At first it was just the flu, but I had a temperature of 104. That went on for a couple of weeks and then my lung collapsed.

That's when the doctors said, "Excuse me, you've got PCP," which totally freaked me out. What the fuck are you telling me here? They were trying to explain how this only happens to certain individuals. Then he started asking questions about my sexuality as far as, "Are you gay?" or "Do you use drugs?" "What the fuck does that have to do with the fact that you came in here and told me that I have pneumonia?" Then he told me he was going to diagnose me with GRID.

I guess it was 1985 when I decided to get tested. Sure enough, it came back positive but my T-cells were like at 800. I was still freaked out because here it is, we're in Texas. You were getting very little information through the news and through the community itself. You still really did not know what HIV was, what GRID was, and what all that meant. Having to be lying there flat on your back in 1983 with doctors and nurses looking like astronauts coming into your room, not able or willing to touch you, not wanting to do things for you is probably the most humiliating thing for a human being to feel. You get totally freaked out. What the fuck? Here I was already living with a man for the last ten years so it's like, what does this mean to me?

My lover was pissed off at the fact that I had received this diagnosis of GRID. How is it spread? Can we get it by touching? Can we get it by kissing? I mean, all that stuff ran amuck among your head. How it was going to play out? Kurt, my lover, was so pissed off with me and so mad. It was more what I was given so to speak or the diagnosis that was given to me. He was flat out scared at the fact that here I was, owner of two restaurants. People find out you're queer. People find out you got GRID or AIDS, there goes your business. There were rumors around that you could get it from waiters that were serving food. It took a toll on you of not knowing what was true and what wasn't and whether you were going to die today or in five minutes. The doctors told me flat out in the hospital that I had five months. Goodbye. I had been so stressed out since '83 and here it is '85, what is this all about?

Beyond having no idea . . .

John Cailleau I got tested for curiosity more than anything else. But it must have been that they had some idea that it had something to do with sexual activity. I figured that since I had been incredibly sexually active there was at least the possibility that I had this whatever it was that was causing this weird disease. So I went to an anonymous testing site at 17th near Castro, got tested, had some bureaucratic counselor talk with me after she gave me the results. When she told me I was positive, I handled it incredibly well right there. I wasn't a mess or all that surprised. When I got home all of it hit me.

John pulls out a tape labeled, "DEPRESSED" from when he tested positive for HTLV-3 and puts it in the tape machine. A barely audible angry voice emerged from the fuzz of the decade-old recording: "Now lets see what I can say about myself tonight 'cause I feel like shit. This afternoon I got a positive antibody notice which doesn't mean anything except that it's possible for me to get AIDS. It means I probably am contagious and can transmit it and I know I got about a 20 percent odds of coming down with it, an 80 percent odds of not coming down with it. I feel like something fucking went off in my stomach tonight."

John trails off about a number of problems: "Now let's talk about me being forty-six years old and not having any close personal friends that I do things with, nobody. If I don't go to my parents for Christmas I will probably be alone, one of those orphans nobody wants. Let's talk about me having an ugly nose. Let's talk about nobody being attracted to me. Let's talk about nobody ever calling to go out and do anything with me."

John turns off the tape: As you can see, I was to my ankles and beyond in self-pity. It's pretty evident from the tone that I didn't feel I had a lot of support mechanisms in place. I must have called a couple of friends. At that time, most people didn't know their HIV status. Most people were not even thinking about their own disease status.

Robert Boulanget Phillip was the type that never whined. We worked together and he complained being tired. He always had been. Then he had a boil on his leg that wouldn't cure and he had to go to the doctor to have it all cut out because it got infected. Then he started not being well and things happened very fast. I think they did happen a lot faster back then because we didn't have all this knowledge yet. This was at the beginning. He always had a hunger pain, like when you get hungry. The doctors tested and tested until finally they found KS in his stomach. I think as he got sicker he began to accept his dependencies.

Darnell Davis I remember a friend coming out to visit in L.A. and saying to me, "Are you positive or negative?" I had no idea what the fuck he was talking about. We, here on the West Coast, didn't know. It took us a long time to even understand what the boys on the East Coast were going through. It first hit me when my friend went to New York. He went to the hospital with the flu and he was dead. That's absurd. There's got to be more to it than that. When it did come to us on the West Coast, it was something that we didn't think about. It was total ignorance. I was too busy working and having a good time. Then all of a sudden, slowly, people you knew were gone. We were all going through denial. Nobody wanted to get tested. I guess all of us who didn't get tested right away probably knew that we were already infected. It was hard to finally wake up and realize that this is real.

Philip Blazer I remember hearing friends say, "Oh, I would kill myself if I found out I was positive." Testing was the thing to do. It was something everyone talked about. The test had just come out.

I got my results on November 13, 1986. I remember I was shopping at Macy's that day. There was a big sale and it's like, "I don't want to go get my test, that's gonna be less time I have for shopping," and I almost didn't go. I was all a hop and skip and a jump. I think I had smoked a little pot. I was heading down Castro to Market to take the underground and go shopping. I thought, "Well, I have a little extra time, let me go over to the Health Department to get my results," and I was floored. I was in shock. I couldn't believe the news I had just gotten, like no, this isn't me. They counseled a little bit and I went home and called two friends and they were both supportive.

I thought of my grandfather who actually passed away. I went to see him before I left 'cause I knew it would be a while before I got back. He said, "Well, all my friends, everybody I ever knew went to California ended up dying." (*Laughs.*) That's the first thing I thought of; that stuck with me. I finally get to a point where I am so happy, where I am so elated.

I still get goose bumps when I go out sometimes. I get out here and get established and bam, this has to happen.

Paul Greenbaum   Gradually, I've evolved more into gay culture but at the time I was diagnosed, my gay life was primarily the various friends I made and going to the bars or the baths. Basically I was very naive about gay life. After the AIDS epidemic arose, I started watching Reagan and becoming informed about the politics and the organizations. I knew, if anyone would be HIV-positive, it would be me.

In '85, '86 I started becoming aware. The point was driven home. I had a long distance fling. You don't always think these things will pan out, but his big hang-up was that he was negative and I had not taken the test. There was still no treatment. He did not want to go forward. "Yes, I'll still love you if you are positive," he claimed but I knew.

Around September, October of '86, I started developing KS spots and I knew deep down what all that was. The next few months were spent trying to come to terms with this intellectually before I finally decided to just do it. I went to the doctor and said what I thought. I had had a couple of other problems. I had had what we later learned were hairy leucoplakia, the growth on the inside of your tongue, recurrent herpes outbreaks. As I started reading about AIDS related issues, I read that oral hairy leukoplakia was an early sign of immune suppression. It was an opportunistic infection, although not a disabling form. The facts were starting to fall into place.

Time bombs, part two – health insurance

David Pattent   In the meantime, I moved into the house. Bill gets out of the hospital. They basically have told him that he, too, is dying, that he needs to get his affairs in order, and that they're going to try and medically retire him. I had started working at another travel agency in Las Vegas and befriended this woman Jeanine. During our dialoguing I tell her this whole story, not realizing this woman's a complete schizophrenic and she has called the Health Department of Las Vegas, saying that Bill and I are spreading the gay plague amongst the community. The Health Department didn't act on it. What they did do is call to tell the Base Commander that Bill and I were being promiscuous and spreading this virus around. So there was another red flag over Bill's head. So now we've got the homosexual issue, the GRID issue, and the promiscuity issue with the OSI looking at all of this stuff. And eventually we got busted. We spent a great deal of the rest of the decade in and out of court battling with the military over Bill's dishonorable discharge. Ten years in the military and no disability.

October of '84, we moved to Gainesville where Bill was going to teach. Bill applies for the GI Bill, and the Veteran's Administration says, "No, we can't fund you because you're a person who's dying from this disease." That's when we found out that he was only rated for the 10 percent disabled by the Veteran's Administration, "You're dying, but you're only 10 percent disabled. And you're not really sick enough that we can rate you at a hundred percent disabled."

During that Gainesville period, in January of 1985, Bill got real sick. I called the SAMs. Bill had this severe ear infection and a temperature of about 103. There was a Veteran's Administration hospital right next to the Teaching Hospital. I took him to the emergency room and it essentially took eighteen hours for him to be seen, because he was rated at 10 percent disabled. Even though he was running a fever of 103, was delirious, couldn't stand up. It took me about ten hours to secure a gurney for him to lie down on. The hospital did not want to hear. They did not want to know about his problems. So, we then take on the Veteran's Administration again. Oh, it was horrible, absolutely horrible, it was hideous, absolutely hideous. We've been fighting for three years at this point. And we never resolved this.

Jay Segal It was frightening. I kept losing jobs over this. I'm one of those stupid people who are honest. If they ask things on forms I answer them truthfully. Actually, when you talk about medical, I would say I was reported to be diagnosed with multiple sclerosis in 1981. That usually kept me out. I was uninsurable for that reason. And everywhere I've worked was a group policy so they had to let me go because I was uninsurable. I hate this virus. I hate what it causes the society to do to those people. You fear the unknown.

Robin Tichane I thought there was a great deal to be lost by finding out: 1) there was no treatment or whatever, so finding out there was no payoff in terms of a treatment, and 2) I was self-employed at the time and there are all kinds of insurance things that might hinge on that. You could be penalized very clearly in terms of medical records by having the test done. So I had no interest in that at all. That was a real conscious decision after watching lots of friends. They had lots of problems and negative side effects. What's the payoff after discovery? By that time everyone was practicing safe or safer sex. So I didn't get tested until '87 and I'd gotten a job at the museum. I thought, well I should probably know. I thought, I have a city job and I can get insurance through them and I'll have health coverage. And AZT might have come up then. I wasn't gangbusters to try it, but I was open to the idea that there might be an upside to this, so I did it. I had a private disability practice and a private life insurance policy. When I was self-employed, for years I had a disability insurance policy which might have been maybe $1,500 a month for life if I'm disabled, and I had a hundred thousand dollar life insurance policy. And funny thing, both get canceled. Hmm, isn't that curious? I got the diagnosis in January of '88. It's supposed to be confidential tests, fuck that. By accident, my worst fears came true. I retired a year later in January of '89. At that point, the health service of the city and county tried to cancel my health insurance. I was just, you sons of bitches, thanks a lot. So I hire an attorney and I go through hell and finally get to keep it and they turn around and triple the price. That's the health service system.

So here I am here, end of '89. I'm trying to put it all together and am fully disabled. I could use that $1,500 for every month for the rest of my life. I could use $100,000 when I die to cover my estate. And I could have used health insurance at one-third of the cost. So it was like society saying we're really going to ostracize you; we're going to mark you; you're going to be punished. To this day the insurance companies can cancel both disability and life insurance policies. There are no laws against that and there are laws with lots of loopholes about health insurance coverage. That was my story and, you know, I survived.

Dan Vojir I was finally formally diagnosed in '84. We went to the Health Center One in Castro. I thought it would be absolutely impossible for me not to be. I was ready for a positive diagnosis. I wasn't going to sugar coat it. So, when this guy had to tell me, I calmed him down. I says, "It's OK. Don't worry about it. Forget it." (*Laughing.*) I considered myself a survivor and I was going to just live through the best of it.

Hiding away from the world

G'dali Braverman I did the work, I think, from '82 to '83, and then I took a hiatus from '83 to '88, really. I stepped out of the world, I think, in a different way than most people did. I think a lot of people just sort of took to hiding in hopes that . . . It was like the Jews in Egypt putting lambs' blood on their door so that God would pass over their doors and not smite their first born type thing. I think there was that attitude. If I don't go out and I don't interact then it won't happen.

83

The critical personal point was that my spouse, who I met in '83, became ill and died very quickly. That really changed my perspective on the epidemic and of the gay community. There was so little support. The network was so nonexistent inside of GMHC. The phobia was so thick that you could just cut it with a knife. Most of our friends disappeared or just never came to the hospital and I was at that point, once he was hospitalized, of literally living at the hospital. I had a bed there and I would go to work from the hospital in the morning and come back directly after five o'clock and live there . . . We were kids and we didn't expect that this was going to be part of our lives. We knew this was going to be part of our life but not our lives as young men. He was twenty-two, so the future was ours, but that's the way the cards fell.

Paul Greenbaum In March of '87 I went to the doctor and they did a biopsy on the lesions and yes, it was KS. I thought I was through. I actually did my will before I went to the doctor. And, yes, that's what it was. I went through a lot of depression and helplessness after I got the official diagnosis. I pretty much crawled into this room and this opens up (*gesturing to the couch we're sitting on*) and I actually stayed in this room. I didn't do like Yoko Ono did after John Lennon was assassinated, crawl into her bed and have people bring her things and never come out of the bedroom or open the blinds.

Hank Wilson There was a period of several years when people shut down. People were terrified. We knew there was a problem. And because you don't know how to maneuver through this, it just freaked everybody out. People were learning about what AIDS was; you would see people on the street who knew that they had it. It was a horrible thing to go from seeing people and then seeing people who are sick.

Peter Groubert But, as the '80s started going along, after '82, say '83, '84, more and more people were getting sick. Fear was gripping the city and the nation. Gay people stopped going out. Nobody knew how it was transmitted and people were afraid. The dance clubs started closing, lots of restaurants went belly-up. There used to be lots more neighborhood movie theaters, the El Ray and stuff. They all went under. In the beginning I cried and I went to all the memorials. I forgave everyone all their transgressions against me. And it tore me up. These were people my age. It was frightening. Here, I thought that I had this bug and I pretty much knew it even though I didn't actually, and people were dying. Well, from '82 to '86 I stayed at home. I became a hermit. I basically waited to die. I ended relationships. I gave away a lot of my possessions and I was preparing to die.

States of clusterfuck

Philip Blazer It then progressed to a state of, I use this term a lot, a state of clusterfuck. It was information overload. All of a sudden there was nothing and then there was just all this information. What do you do? Who do you see? Should I be taking this? Drink the water, or not, everywhere you turned, there was all this information.

PART III

Death

SEVEN

Bearing Witness to the Dying

As the plague earned a formal name, AIDS, and began taking thousands of victims, Los Angeles, New York and San Francisco became the disease epicenters. During the early years, San Franciscans had to live with both the difficult reality of an incurable illness and a healthy world in ignorance only selectively observing the epidemic. For many, the close association with friends and lovers as they died became a call to arms. "It's where we learn about love, where we discover new values and qualities in ourselves. Death joins sex as a community sublime," Robert Gluck puts it. However, this didn't happen overnight. Many turned away from community life. Bob Lee took on visiting those left behind in the hospitals. As he took care of his dying lover, Darnell found a new approach to his own life. For G'dali, taking care of his spouse as he died served as a call to political action. After the losses of his best friend and partner to AIDS, Allan Troxler put AIDS and its relationship to the American political landscape into a proper context: "I see now why Whitman embraced the chance to nurse Civil War soldiers. Surely the democracy of death confirmed all the egalitarian effusion of *Leaves of Grass*."

Ronnie Ashley Aside from the money, the politics, the agencies, the bottom line still remains with us, our responsibility as people to take care of our family and our people. There's something that happens to individuals when you go from being an independent person to a disabled individual and can no longer take care for yourself and you've lost control of your bowels. You become very humbled and your priorities change. Your way of thinking about life changes. How do we deal with it? There ain't no manual written about the terminally ill. Everything is different.

Bob Lee *Bob Lee's lover died in their home in '87. He shared recollections of the loneliness he felt in a community that had gone into hiding.* For a long time I would not go and visit anybody in the hospital after the experience. I really resented all his friends who never came by the house, who never called. Now I'm starting to have compassion for them, but I didn't for a long time. I couldn't do it. It's so hard. I can do it now. God did this.

One of my very best friends going back to when I was in Atlanta, Bob, got very sick. I was able to visit Bobby. Every Monday I would go see him at Davies Medical Center. Sunday night at MCC, Metropolitan Christian Church, it just so happened that the rector from St. Johns was doing the visitation that night. One of Bob's chief caregivers was there. He was saying, "You know, he's dying. He's not going to make it through the night." And the rector says, "Bob would you come with me?"

So I went to the hospital with them. It was obvious that Bob was near death. He was not able to talk. He had tubes down his throat and all. Bob's eyes were very, very much alive. And I knew that Bobby could hear what we were talking to him about. And Warren, our rector at the time, starts a caring, loving meditation and was touching him, a letting go kind of meditation. And he had to go.

So while I was still there, I took over when he was done. He did all the rites and that kind of stuff. I sat on Bobby's bed and he had TB so I had to wear the mask and all that stuff. There was so little of his body that I could touch physically, just sort of rubbed his arm with my left hand like I was petting my cat, just a loving touch. I had my hand right on his heart where I could feel his heart beating. I just started talking to Bobby 'cause I knew he could hear me. And I started talking about this past life together, how many wonderful experiences we had. For a letting go type of meditation I said, "It's OK Bobby. Die. That's what you have to do. It's OK. You know, we'll miss you. Our love will go with you. That doesn't die. Your daughter is going to hurt. She's going to miss you but you'll still be there for her. It's OK Bobby."

This, I don't know if you want it on the tape or not. Part of Bobby's and my experiences over the years were in fist-fucking and speed and whatever. My inner voice just brought this out when I realized what a struggle Bobby was having fighting death. He was really fighting it. Actually I says, "Bobby, remember the first time a man ever put his fist up your butt? How much it hurt when he started and how wonderful it was when you just relaxed and let it in and how marvelous that felt." I could see the smile in his eyes. "Just think how wonderful it will be when you just open your body and let God come in and let him take you home with him to where you belong." And very shortly after that Bobby's breathing was very shallow and very rapid. He took one deep breath. My hand was still on his chest. I could feel his heart beating. He took one deep breath and he held it in for a second. And he let it out and I could feel his heart slowing down. He took a second deep breath and he just went "hhhhh," so beautiful and so peaceful. And I felt the last beat of his heart. It was so beautiful and so peaceful sharing the death with this man, seeing him make that transition. And I sat there just holding him and sending him my love for at least five minutes before I went out and got the nurse. The nurses at Davies are so wonderful. If I had known I would have been the person in there when Bob died I would have run so far in the other direction. I would have flown to Arizona if I had had to. It was almost exactly 1:20 in the morning when he took his last heartbeat. I walked up to the nurses' desk and all of a sudden this rage just came after me. It must have been almost two in the morning and I screamed at the top of my lungs and just pounded the nurses' station, "GOD DAMN THIS FUCKING DISEASE!" And a nurse got up from her station, puts her arms around me and says, "Rob, let's just take you back here. You can rest." She took me back to the head nurse's private office, sat me down, said, "There's the phone. Make any calls you need to make. If they are long distance, don't worry about it. The hospital can afford it." And she brought a cup of coffee.

Darnell Davis *Darnell found a man who showed him how to live on in this world with AIDS.* I was always single, independent. I knew he was also HIV-positive. He had just lost a lover a couple years prior. We met on a Friday night when I didn't want to go out but I was dragged out anyway, and we were together from that day forth. He taught me that it was OK. He taught me that it was important to care about oneself. At that point I still didn't go to a doctor. This was a couple of years even later. I just would not go. He tricked me. I had an earache, so we went to the doctor. He says, "Tell the doctor you're HIV-positive." So I did. And he was sittin' in the waiting room laughing 'cause I was back there for three, four fuckin' hours. And I came out and said, "You little fucker, you knew they were going to do this to me" which was good because he used to be a registered nurse. I thank him to this day for doing that for me, that just showing how much he cared; and he made me start caring too. That's when I started educating myself.

Until then I tried to pretend like it wasn't a big thing when in turn, deep down in my soul, it was tearing me apart. At age twenty, a friend asked, "Why are you so self-destructive?" I went to therapy and I realized I was angry with my mom, sixteen years later. A four-year-old going to his mother's funeral and not being told a damn thing knows a hell of a lot more than people give him credit for. I knew I was never going to see her again. I lost my dad when I was seventeen; I lost a sister. It's been hard.

No one wants to wake up one day and know that your time is limited. I had planned on being sixty or seventy, a dirty old man, but I don't think that's going to happen. And then again it may. You know? It was something I had not planned on. To me, my lover was something that was brought to me for a reason. It's funny, we met and we talked about our HIV status the first night. When we went into this relationship, we knew this. We also knew that we were going to be together regardless. We didn't know how much time either of us had. We didn't know if I was going to get sick or if he was going to get sick or what. It just happened that he got sick first, out of the blue.

For a year and a half after that I did nothing but take care of him. I quit work; he was the most important thing to me. People respected me for that. My family respects me for that, and it made me grow up a lot. I thought I was an adult but, after this, I think I've covered all bases. In between accepting the fact and denial, I realized that we were going to get through this, but I was going to come out alone. But I didn't come out alone.

Robert Boulanget *Robert nursed two lovers, Phillip and Tom, before they died. He pets his cat, looks out his fifth-story panoramic view of Market Street and recalls past years of lives he used to share, now faded. In a calm, Quebec accent Robert remembered Phillip's last days.* He just liked to be home and to listen to music instead of going out. The last few days, he kept on getting up and walking and I couldn't control him. His mother stayed in Sacramento. I took care of him until he died. He was blind in one eye. "I want to sleep in the front room," he said. He wanted to move. Maybe he was looking for oxygen. So I called the nurse and she says, "Well, maybe you should get oxygen." The guy came with the truck and I said, "I don't want that in my house." Some people might say how horrible but I didn't want him to have a gas mask on and this big orange tank in the corner. I didn't think it was dignified. I sent it back and called the hospice nurse and said, "Did you hear what I did?" And she said, "That's fine. Whatever you think. You're the doctor." That was nice. That felt natural to me. 'Cause he had been in the hospital and told me to get him out of there. I didn't want any tubes. And that has changed too. I'm sure that patients go in there and say, "I don't want all that crap. I just want to be comfortable." It was all automatic. They went in there and when you came out they'd put the tube down your throat. It just overwhelms you. It becomes everything.

Once you accept that you are going to die, go on that way and forget about this way. I always said, if you give into it, it will be fine and it was. I kept telling Phillip, "God, you love science fiction. This is the ultimate science fiction." His mother kept saying, "When you die, it's like hitting a fly on the wall." She just didn't have the same spirituality as I do. Somehow I think it's more, it's something.

Phillip died real fast; I gave him a shot of morphine. I had to give him morphine shots every three or four hours. That was the hardest thing. I couldn't do it. I would have to talk myself into it. There was no more place to prick him, he was so skinny. I think he died very peacefully, all-in-all. I realized I was spiritual in watching him.

The morning he died, I put the curtains up and played Pink Floyd, "Welcome to the Machine" and "Shine on Your Crazy Diamond" from *Wish You Were Here*, and "The Four Seasons" loud on these speakers. The tenants upstairs knew he had died. It was for me. It's hard not feeling relieved after going through what you've gone through and to know that he is where he is meant to be. God, you've got to understand that.

One night, a month before he died, I said, "Phillip, don't you think we should have that talk?" And he says, "What talk?" And I said, "You know, there must be a talk that people have to do before they die, I guess." And he said, "No, we don't have to have the talk. I wrote you a note I want you to read after I am gone." He died October 30th, '85.

I managed to let myself be hit but I didn't fall down. Then I got diagnosed. After seeing your lover wither, nothing could be worse. I wasn't afraid of dying anymore. Life isn't always that great. After Phillip I thought, if I get three years then if I die that'll be OK.

One Sunday morning, this was probably December, a month and a half later, when it was raining and it was really sad I looked at all the pictures and thought, this Sunday, I really need it and opened that envelope. It just said, "I just wanted you to know that I love you," which he had never said to me all those years. I thought, "Wow, really, why didn't you tell me?" Then it said, "Find a friend and be happy. See you on the other side." And, of course, it was the cries and it was comforting. I'm glad he did that. It made me very happy, well, happy and unhappy, it's all very mixed feelings. That's all life was back then, AIDS always took precedence, overshadowing everything. You couldn't do anything. It was always there, always, always, always.

Starting to live again

It wasn't long after that that I heard about the first group for people who are HIV-positive. John Kraus had lost his lover Frank Laborko. These guys were very talented. They had built a house up on a hill there, took a Victorian and redid it into a modern palace. It was just fabulous. One was a designer and one was an architect. Frank had died and John realized that he knew a lot of people around him who had lost their lovers and there was no support group for lovers. He decided to start a group spontaneously called the Mary Widows.

I went back to Montreal trying to look back for my old self 'cause I didn't know who I was after Phillip died. I was lost. I had been living other people's lives. I had no life so I had to create one for myself. Luckily that's what saved me. I started really living after I came back. Joining that group of The Widows and listening to other people's stories, I realized that I wasn't the only one who had a story like mine with Phillip's mother. Other people had problems with relatives. It seemed like it was inevitable. This one guy was telling that his lover's relatives came. He was the lover and they treated him like shit. They had to have statues and candles burning and the priest coming every day and having masses in the room. All the things that his lover needed his mother just did not want. There was nothing he could do or say. He was just lost there. And he could only see him at certain times.

People kept saying, what do you like the most. I said plants. They said well maybe that's what you should do. From then on things started happening. It seemed like whatever I wanted I was able to fulfil like I had somebody watching over me. Before Phillip died I was always afraid of everything – getting hit by a car, being stabbed. Then, once you're not afraid of death I think it clears up a lot of your other phobias. It wasn't an easy go. Nothing is. I like a lot of the drama of it.

Tom

'91 is when I met Tom. I had met a few other people, not too many. I used to go to the gym a lot, every morning, right down the street at Muscle System. Tom looked like a dancer. He walked like a dancer. He was very truly androgynous, very effeminate and very masculine, an angelic look. He didn't talk to too many people but one morning he said, "You got a haircut." I started talking and one thing led to another; he said that he was a gardener and I said I was a gardener.

After I met Tom, I started helping him with the gardening and we became very close. He told me that he was HIV-positive and we started spending a lot of time together. We would spend long evenings listening to music, painting watercolors by candlelight and drinking a bottle of wine and smoking a little pot. It got to be very comfortable.

He started being in pain a few weeks later. Then I took him to the Emergency. Now, they are opening a new clinic on Saturdays and Sundays for AIDS crisis so people don't have to go through Emergency anymore. It was horrible, simply was horrible. It took forever. First they take you from waiting to this one room where everyone is on gurneys. They don't do very much but assess what you have. He was very afraid. The worst thing about being sick is when you don't know what you have, that stuff frightens. It's the unknown. Anyways, the four o'clock crew came. It was getting busy. There were crazy people tied up. San Francisco General, in Emergency you see everything.

They thought he had TB but they didn't know. They went in there and they thought he had fluid in his lungs. They never knew what it was. He had fluid in his lungs until he died. Weird, you had to wear masks to go in and see him. Of course I didn't wear a mask.

He would go to the bathroom and he says, "I don't know what's wrong. I just can't do it. I know I have to go." The urologist didn't know what he had. But they give him a catheter and told him that's what he should do. He was upset. I would be too. So they decided to send him to this doctor at UC Med which was supposed to be incredible. He had fifteen minutes. He was told, "You have that much time with the doctor. If you come in late the minutes just go away. You have to tell him everything." He didn't show me anything. I'm very difficult for him, I guess. I want to have some kind of a rapport with the doctor. I don't want him to be just a technician in a white suit with gloves. I want him to be a human being that is not afraid to look me in the eye. You know, I don't want a pat on the back either. I want a connection.

Tom's brother was a hospice nurse, a nurse who takes care of dying people. And his brother was gay and Tom had never mentioned his brother until one day he said, "Oh, my brother is coming to visit." Finally, it was like, "And he's gay." It was like he was ashamed. I thought, God, your brother is gay, you never told me.

Tom was on morphine when he came home after seeing that one doctor for fifteen minutes. They did an MRI and realized that some of the brain had been damaged by HIV. I guess that started explaining away what was happening. During all that time we still painted and we still listened to music. And then one day this French woman was singing a song. He asked me to translate that one. He says, "What does this song mean?" Then I said, "Just a minute," and when the refrain came I said, as I was saying it I was realizing what I was saying, "There was this bird. Somebody cut their wings." Then he started crying and said, "That's the way I feel." And I think for that instant I think he felt like he was in bed and that was it. What a horrible feeling that must be? It must be devastating to know that you have no more wings. We don't realize what it's like to be able to walk from here to the bathroom.

So I started crying and I was crying like I've never cried. I don't cry very often so when I cry, I cry for Phillip, for everything. Tom was in bed, he grabbed me, and hugged me and really comforted me and it was OK. That's what I wanted with Phillip that I never had. And when I asked him, "Should we have that talk?" I wanted to cry in his arms and say, You're dying. But we never had that so I never felt that.

Death and America

His brother would call but I wasn't allowed to tell Tom it was him. Tom would say, "God, my brother hasn't called. He said he was going to call." He was doing things behind his back. It was like he couldn't face it. That's the story of all those people, Phillip's mother and all, that is they can't face it. Maybe it's too fast for them to face it right away.

Then, his two brothers from Ohio came to visit. They hadn't seen Tom in a long time and didn't know about him. A lot of us gay people have gone away from our families. We didn't stay home because they treated us like we were something out of this world so we came here. All of a sudden the family drops in because somebody is dying. I never understood why they didn't do it until before. But they always came.

His two brothers were both straight. They didn't know much about him but they were very warm, real nice to me. They spent some time with Tom and some time with me. I showed them the city. The fact that I was there with Tom made them feel good. But they didn't know what was happening with Tom. Tom wasn't coherent.

An acquaintance of David's called. They were both hospice nurses. She said, "I am a friend with so and so and I am running early. Would you mind if I come by now?" It was exactly what I needed, someone to talk to. She knew that at that stage what most people forget is the caregiver. She said, "How are you?" I said, "Fine," but I started crying and I said, "I don't know what to do and David is a hospice nurse and I was taking

care of Tom. Now he comes over and moves him on the count of three."
It was 1, 2, 3. God, I hated that. I said, "He stopped his morphine." She
said, "He did? Oh God." I said, "I think it's because his parents are
coming and he wants him to be coherent." She said, "Well, families
shouldn't take care of their patients. I always tell my customers, Sedated
and Comfortable or Not-Sedated but in pain all the time."

And the Friday morning I met the mother and looked in her eyes. I
truly saw all the pain of all the mothers. I really felt it. Once you meet
the mother, that's the moment of truth. So I hugged her and kissed her
and started crying and crying. I said, "It's not fair," and she said, "Well,
we've been doing a lot of that lately." But she was smiling.

We spent Saturday night with "the family." Everybody was there. Tom
said it had been horrible but "It's part of the dance." I remember him
saying he had to live that as part of the dying process. Apparently, during
the night he tried to die. He said, "I think they wanted me to die." He
said something. "I wanted to die for them and I couldn't do it."

The night before when I was at my friend's house, I remember calling
in the middle of the night, dreaming. I said, "Phillip just died," (*in a
whisper*) and then I woke up and hung up thinking, "What am I doing?"
There were too many parallels between the two and it was too much,
really hitting me.

I used to give him baths and he was so constipated that nothing would
come out with the morphine. It had been days and days and days and he
was in pain because of it. It was very painful. I finally decided to douche
him, but only some of it would come out. Finally I just had to put my
fingers in there and get it out myself because it was completely blocked.
He was in pain but it made him feel better. You could tell that he was
relieved but I could not believe what I was doing. It was so overwhelming
that it was like I was watching a movie with somebody else doing it. When
he was laying in the bathtub I had to let the water go off while he was
still in there because I didn't want him to get cold. He was so thin I could
see the water just sitting inside the skin of his collar bones. I remember
seeing that vividly. Not long after that, he went to the hospital and I never
saw him again.

Bill's death

David Pattent Bill died on October the 24th, 1989. Actually a very, very
amazing experience. I can't view it in anything but a positive light. Bill and
I had always been very realistic about the fact that one of us was going to

go. We didn't know who was going to go first. Towards the end, round about 1987, we both realized that it was probably going to be Bill. It was real important for Bill to know that no matter what happened, I was going to be all right. So we even went to a point of picking out a home that I was going to buy before he died ...

He went into the hospital the first time in 1989. That was the first really big bout. He had PCP. He was in the hospital for about five weeks. During that period of time we realized, OK, we're running out of time now. I stopped working for the international designer and Bill and I just started spending as much time as we possibly could together, going on little vacations. He lost a tremendous amount of weight; he was like this little Ethiopian person. It was like quiet resignation. We both knew that he was dying and that we had to spend as much time as we could together, doing the things that we liked to do. Just laying on the ocean, and we lived by the water so it was real easy for us to do that. Low key stuff. We loved to have dinner parties, so we would have three or four a week. During dinner it was always customary for Bill to go take a nap, for an hour and a half. All our friends knew and accepted that about him. It was an amazing experience. It was beautiful; it was sad; it was touching; it was intimate, many emotions but it wasn't negative.

The final straw came in July of 1989. Bill had these really really bad headaches. So we went into the hospital. They did a CAT scan on him, and they couldn't find anything wrong. Well, the headaches started getting worse, so by the end of July, we knew the writing was on the wall. We called his family. Said, "We're sending you all plane tickets, come on down. Let's spend a few weeks together and have a summer vacation together." The whole family converged on us. There were like nine members of his family, including nieces and nephews and the whole gang. We spent a week just existing and having a really nice time. About three days after his family left he had to go back into the hospital again because the headaches had come back and they were getting worse. He was starting to have problems with his speech. The doctor said, "Okay, we need to do an MRI," Magnetic Resonance Imaging. During the MRI they found out he had PML, which is progressive multifocal leukoencephalo-pathy. The doctor was a very good friend of ours and didn't have the nerve to tell Bill. So he told me, "I'm going to leave this up to you to tell Bill that he's dying."

I went into Bill's hospital room and we had a long discussion about the fact that, "Okay this is it. We've known all along that this is going to be a reality at some point and you're going to die, and now it's time to die." He decided he didn't want to die in the hospital. We'd always been very clear that he wanted to die at home. We pulled him out at the end of July. Basically his reaction to me was this: I'd designed a ring (*shows me a ring on his hand*) and given it to him that Christmas. When he came home from the hospital we were in the kitchen and we were just hugging each other and he said, "I guess it's time for me to start dying." And he took the ring off and he slid it onto my finger. At that point I kinda knew that this was it, he had resigned himself. And we both cried a little bit. It was not very dramatic. I'd always envisioned this "Oh, Oh," falling apart and stuff. But it wasn't. It was actually kinda neat, because in his acceptance, I had to move to a place of acceptance of it. That was the only way. We had always been strong for each other.

Then he spent the next three months dying. Slowly but surely all of his faculties started going away from him. I had to assume the responsibility for care of his body. We'd always had a pact that when the time came, that I would help him go out. July, August, September, he became weaker and weaker. I used to have to start brushing his teeth, shaving him. We started out in the shower with him on a bar stool. We had a plastic cover over the bar stool and I would hold him while I bathed him in the shower. Then that couldn't work any more after about a few weeks. So then we moved him into this big Roman tub. And we just spent all this time doing amazing closure stuff. I didn't realize, but when I reflect back on it, it's like that was a really beautiful experience, because we were able to say goodbye to one another in such an intimate way that under normal circumstances wouldn't have happened had we gone into it with the drama aspect of it. We didn't do the drama aspect. We did it as this is something that's happened, we know it's going to happen, and let's do this the best way that we know how to do it. Slowly but surely he became weaker and weaker. Eventually he got to the point he couldn't leave the bed.

He lost his vision; he went blind. And basically you lose all of your abilities to function. He got to a point where he could no longer talk. So I started doing – I'd ask him questions, you know, "Raise your finger once if for yes and raise your finger twice if for no." He had always said to me that when it got to the point where he could no longer communicate or function in his body, that I had to stop feeding him. About two weeks before he lost his speech, we had the discussion that that time was coming. And three weeks before he died, I had to make the decision to stop feeding him. I asked him. I said, "Bill, do you want to eat?" and he slowly lifted two fingers. So I stopped feeding him and he started going downhill very rapidly. At that point in time, I'd brought hospice in, only because I knew that's where I could get the drugs that I needed to kill him. Basically that's what I did. I essentially took Bill's life for him. He died in my arms at about three in the morning.

I did everything that I possibly could to make him as comfortable as possible. And spent the last two or three days just talking to him, letting him know how much I loved him, recounting the experiences we had gone through, the things we had done. Going down memory lane, almost like a mental photo album. And then he died very peacefully in my arms at about three o'clock in the morning. I was with him for about two or three hours before I called the mortician. And just prepped his body, washed his hair for the first time in four or five days, brushed his teeth, put his partial back in because he wore a partial. When they came to pick him up he was dressed, his hair was combed. Everything was done. He was just laying there very peacefully. I went outside and they removed his body. That was the last I saw of him.

I was in the mind set of "Oh my God, I'm going to die next." That to me was like a reality alert. I went traveling to visit friends. Not depressed. I wasn't in a space of "Woe is me, I just lost my lover." It's just like, What am I going to do between now and the time I die? And six months pass and then nine months passed and my immune system went to 2002. (*Laughs.*) God knows what was going on but I realized, I wasn't going anywhere. The notion of me dying got real boring. So I started work again and to come out to California. And here I am today. I've met another wonderful human being, Neil, at an AIDS research program in South Africa. He was the most successful import I did.

EIGHT

Room for Loss

As the years of the epidemic continued, issues surrounding the impact of death and bereavement on both people with AIDS and the uninfected accumulated. The expression, "Not Infected, Affected" relates to this. Many faced the reality of having lost five, ten, or hundreds of friends, lovers, and colleagues to the disease. Some, many of whom came to San Francisco with the '70s migration, watched an entire social circle from old college roommates to best friends and acquaintances be decimated. "There was a feeling that I am going to be the last one here to turn out the lights," one PWA observed (Garfield and Spring, 1993).

Kübler-Ross (1969, 1987) suggests that people go through stages of grief when there is a loss. Healing occurs when people undergo these stages. If the process is interrupted, not once but on many occasions, then the bereaved individual does not heal from loss. In a treatise on reviving community mental health, Rofes (1996: 5) writes: "Many of us have reached the stage of the epidemic where we have reached the limitation of our ability to mourn. When I look deeply into myself, I find evidence that normal cycles of grief are not occurring." This phenomenon, comparable to post traumatic stress syndrome, has been labeled multiple loss syndrome (MLS) (Grothe and McKusick, 1993). MLS, often manifesting itself in a form of clinical depression related to loss (Grossman and Silverstein, 1993; Moynihan et al., 1988; Neugenebauer et al., 1992; Chrysler, 1995), commands an inordinate social impact for those affected by the epidemic.

Both Grothe and McKusick (1993) and Neugenebauer et al. (1992) concur that continued involvement within community and personal life help reduce depression around loss. San Francisco proved a dynamic community for gay men and lesbians before AIDS. When the epidemic hit, the city responded (Fernandez, 1991). Opportunities for continued community involvement for PWAs became a primary component of the San Francisco response to the epidemic. As Robert Boulanget explained, his participation within the Mary Widows within months of his lover's death played a key role in his quest to start to live again.

Dr. Charles Garfield's (see Garfield and Clark, 1978; Garfield, 1978, 1995) Shanti Project, a volunteer counseling outfit since 1974, adapted its goals and brought volunteers through two-week trainings to prepare to become caregivers for PWAs. Successes, however, were relative.

Eric Rofes (1996), the former director of Shanti Project, views multiple loss theory as limited in its capacity to address the needs of those enduring the inevitable psychic numbing resulting from participation within a death saturated community life (pp. 15–42). He suggests that fresh approaches, including the use of narrative theory (p. 75), are needed to mend "the fabric of gay community life" (p. 89).

Experience with multiple loss changes people, cities (such as San Francisco), and cultures. AIDS has led to a new national reckoning with death and disease (Rich, 1995; Nuland, 1994; Moller, 1995). Interviewees talk about their lessons from loss and their attempts to find spaces within their psyches for memories of those who are gone. Some interviewees reflect MLS, others insights into a new reality, and most combinations of both.

Nancy Lemoins   *I first got to know Nancy at the Shanti House. We met at Josie's Cabaret for our interview. Her hair is medium short; she wears white shorts and a T-shirt without sleeves revealing tanned swimmer's shoulders from constant bike riding, and a silver pendant for serenity. She told me about the days in the Seattle lesbian underground of the '70s:* I was a teamster. That's when I was doing a lot of drugs because I had so much money but I was this hippie. My rent was like $200. I bicycled everywhere I went and I was painting and really happy. I was such a radical, such an incredibly political person. Then Reagan got elected in 1980. It was just I had no belief that he was going to win and I just was so shocked. I was like I can't believe this is happening. We gotta go. It was very political and very idealistic. I had spent a year in Paris in college. My girlfriend and her ex-boyfriend at the time decided that we should move to Paris.

Between that 1980 trip and the present, worlds disappeared. She elaborated on trying to find room, psychological space for the memories of all those friends. I have this photograph of when I was in seventh grade. I had this best friend, his name was Jeffrey and when he came back from a trip to New York between seventh and eighth grade, he told me he was gay. I said I knew I was too and we were like best friends in eighth grade. It was a very interesting friendship because we were little kids but we thought we were grownups. He was a close friend of mine my whole life. I lost touch with him and then I ran into him about four years ago here. Although he was pretty sick, he didn't seem that sick to me. He said to me one day, "Don't worry about the fungus amungus," which is very stupid. But it was because I had a fungus and he had this fungus and I just remember him walking down the street that day. He was always smoking pot and I was really busy. It's really weird that that was the last thing he ever said to me. I really have such strange feelings about that, that he died and like I knew him my whole life. He was this part of my childhood. I don't know; I don't know where to put him in my life, in my memory. I just can't figure it out.

And I also have another friend from my first year of college. He was a gay man. I remember the first time I ever saw him. I looked at him and thought, He is like absolutely the most gorgeous human being I have ever seen; he was so stunning to me. It wasn't like sex but he was so physically beautiful; he took my breath away. I remember approaching him and saying something really stupid like (*laughs*), "Your eyes are so amazing," because they were unlike any other. I remember like him thinking, "Oh, this is like some straight girl who is coming onto me," and how it was like to tell him I knew he was gay and then for him to find out I was gay. Anyway, we were friends for a really long time.

I was really sure that he would never die. He never did anything. He never went to a doctor; he never took one fucking drug. And when he died, I couldn't reconcile that on any level. I really thought he would live forever. Those are the two people I have the hardest time with. Everyone else has come into my life and I knew they were finite. Those were people who have been there forever, way before AIDS even existed; it's so hard for them to leave. You know, it just doesn't fit. I think about them and their relation to me and the things that I went through and how they can do that. It doesn't make any sense. There's a certain shock with other people that you never can't ever get over. I dream about these people a lot, like really a lot.

Evolving attitudes toward death

Rev. Mark Stanger I had this great old, old professor in Rome. This was Fr. Augustino. He would always lecture in the big lecture hall with a big oil painting of St. Augustine over his head. And a lot of it was just a rave and just sort of pious crap. But he said something theological that was very important. He said, "St. Francis was wrong about death! It's not Sister Death, Gentle Sister Death. Death is the enemy to human enterprise, to everything we love and enjoy and we can't domesticate it." That had a big impression on me and it's the same with disease. It's a rip-off. Death is a rip-off. Every funeral you go to people are crying. Something's been stolen and something's been interrupted. Every time lovers kiss goodbye in the morning, it anticipates death. It anticipates that final goodbye. Every separation. St. Benedict told his monks to keep death daily before your eyes. Now you could surround yourself with Day of the Dead images or with bleeding crucifixes or whatever. But it obviously is an urgency about life. It's this balance again. I will decay and die. That's just what we have to deal with and it's not pretty and it's serious. I have to integrate that all the time in my thinking.

Nancy Lemoins I've known so many people that have died lately. I dream about them all the time. I've been present at three pretty clear deaths and I can't ever get those people out of my mind. That's such an intense moment (*laughs*). In a way it is, and in a way it's just like eating breakfast. I know that sounds weird but it's like, oh you're here and then you're not. You're dying and your heart stops and if you think about it too hard, it's really very weird but if you don't think about it it's kind of like you get up, eat a sandwich and then you die.

Ronnie Ashley (*A former Shanti Project case worker.*) So how, during this whole time of working with AIDS and the fact that you've got a lover dying at home, do you deal with multiple death? How do you deal with it as an individual where it's constantly in your face? To me, this isn't just client 222. This is Robert. I've known Robert for three years. That to me is the person who I am and the work that I do. How do you, as an individual, make your play stronger as far as dealing with multiple death? You know, because you consume so much of it and you have the anger that comes with it; you have the frustration; you have that peace. There are just so many entities that happen to one's self as far as death and dying and the need continually to rebuild our extended families. I've got many women who are no longer here in my life, women that were always in my life and they're no longer here. How do you continue to make friends with people? How do you continue to open up your heart and to embrace everyone and to bring people into your family only having six months, whatever the time period is, having to bury them later on? That takes a toll on your psyche, who you are as an individual in your own soul and in your own heart.

A prostitute told me one time, "Once you start to come with your clients, it's time to get out of the business." I am at a point to where I enjoy my passion; I enjoy my anger; I enjoy the fact that I can still cry. Until there comes a time where I can no longer feel and hurt, where I become a soldier of war, then yes, it's time for me to get out. But I pray to the day that that never happens even though as much and as painful as it is to accept and to acknowledge death, there is also something very rewarding in the gifts that you have received while with individuals who were walking on this earth. My strength comes from them, remembering those that have gone before me, what they went through, what their physical pain was like, what their emotions were like, what their endurance was like, what their mental state was like. All those are entities that are part of the puzzle of how we deal as human beings.

Joey Bankow was a twelve-year-old boy who used to do a lot of Shanti's trainings. He was a hemophiliac and that's how he contracted AIDS. Two months after he died, four of the kids passed away. This whole group of hemophiliacs and kids I had worked with at Shanti and through a children's camp that I do went. And then Jeff, this other five-year-old boy who had been HIV-positive all his life, passed away; I was real close to him. I remember sitting at home and I was just crying and crying and Joey came into my dreams. He was saying, "It's OK, everybody is all right." It was OK. Then I get him; I get Jeff; I get Ricky and I get a couple of these other people. They're these visions of them telling me it's OK to let go 'cause everybody is OK.

As individuals, we need to acknowledge the entity death and dying and what that looks like to us as human beings. Otherwise, we're not going to make it. We need to be able to celebrate that life and to acknowledge that people have come before us, even if it's an Indian and my great ancestors, it's their knowledge that continues to continue on the walk that I'm on. I'm doing the things that I feel for a reason. There's a reason why I've been a long-term survivor of HIV. There's a reason for those that have gone before me.

I went to Mexico for El Día de los Muertos, the celebration of the dead, and seeing that in Mexico City, hundreds of thousands of people in the night-time with the candles and the cemeteries that were decorated to the hilt with offerings for the dead from water and wine and cigarettes and food and flowers. There was an amazing relief and acceptance as far as death was concerned and what that looked like. This was celebrating the lives of these individuals.

I thought, wow, this was such a great way to acknowledge the dead, better than the morbid, funeral type, heavy crying type stuff that we always see. Very much, "Santa María, Jesús . . ." (*Smiles and crosses himself.*) "God, Father," and the Catholic and the guilt, rushing down to the shrink . . . I just think it's a fabulous way as far as a ritual, as far as acknowledging and accepting one's death and to let go and to know that stuff we were just saying, spirits and ghosts and witches and goblins and people are not too sure whether they are and whether they are not and visions and so forth. Baby, open up your heart and your spirit and what you believe and whatever comes to you, take it. We fear fear itself. I can't explain my visions of Joey and Ricky and some of my other friends, whether they're dreams, visions, whatever they may be. At that time, they came in at that time and the emotions and letting me know that things was OK and I was OK and it was like, OK. I feel there are all these souls and spirits that continue to guide me, to hold my strength and my passion, my fear, my hurt. Yeah, I think it's all there.

David Pattent The probably ten or fifteen other people whose hands I've held as they made their transition, it looks real peaceful. I've reached the place in my life, where I know relationships never end, they just redefine themselves. So that person who died three weeks ago, Richard, for example, I miss the fact that I can't talk to him, but I can always have an internal dialogue. I know that that person is always going to be a part of my experience, and that can't be taken away from me. Now there's no distance that he's inside my heart. I don't feel loss. As bizarre as it sounds, I think that's part of the way I deal with the shell shock of having lost over 500 friends in the last twelve years.

Neil (*David's lover*) All the dying was like a huge, big, black thing around you. It changes the way you think about death; it's not a Western thing to do because death is something to shove away. Science pushes it away. We try to define it, but when you're in the middle of this you can't do that; you actually have to look at death and say, What about life now? It becomes part of life. Can't avoid it, so he dies.

David Pattent The Big Ugly is just a cultural thing. It's not about where we are specifically as people. I've traveled in the Middle and Far East and death is an embraced thing. Death is a liberation. And yet, here everyone goes into this big comatose state dragging it out; in other parts of the world dying is so embraced, it's encouraged, it's supported, it's a family thing. Death is life; they are not separate from each other, they are one. Working with it redefines priorities, let's put it that way. Pettiness becomes obviously petty. It becomes very apparent each day.

Ronnie Ashley In Birmingham, Alabama, I think that's where I learned the most – at the Black Baptist churches. The music of this people ran chills up my spine, like my own people when I hear them sing and hear the war dances and hear the songs of the dead and the spirits. There's this longing, longing of music and pain and hurt and passion and love of history out of these individuals that were 90 and 100 years old and in their 80s, men and women that you knew came and had lived history on a whole different level.

God knows it's not easy . . . grief

Jay Segal Everybody that's born, in their young years has dreams, aspirations, hopes, places they want to go and be. I luckily did a lot of them before my world was yanked from under me. But from 1981, it's just been one series of catastrophes after another. The more it happens, the sicker I got. I was heavily in depression.

I don't have very many friends, three but one died. I had a problem last week and I picked up the phone. I went to call Bruce because he's a person who I call when I have problems, went to speed dial and realized he's been deleted. You forget that they die. They're still your friends. They're still close. They're just no longer a speed dial. I'm still grieving. I lost two lovers in one week. That's tough. April was hell. I had more catastrophes pile onto each other. There's a part of me that disappeared. The funny part, the guy who makes jokes, he's gone completely. There's pieces left but . . .

Philip Blazer I've gotten news from my mom about family members who have had tragic things happen and I am just like, "Wow, sorry." I don't know what it is. I'm tapped out from emotions. I've been dealing with this for quite a long time especially in this community. I've seen so much, so much suffering. I don't know a person who hasn't lost somebody or a number of people.

Brad Sherbert Well over 200, 270 funerals or maybe close to 280 now. I keep a large social circle and out here there are so many PWAs. I don't know if you remember my friend Vince who used to visit. Well, over the last year and a half we have become just as close as could be and when I first met him he was just as healthy as me. He's in a bedridden state now. I bet he don't last two more weeks. No matter how many times you see that happen to people, you never get used to it. I was reading an article on multiple loss syndrome. They said when you lose a close friend or something, you need six months to recover. They said since the beginning of the epidemic in Los Angeles, it isn't uncommon for a gay man to have lost fifty friends, they think that is the average, and they talked about the psychological effects of that. What would they think about 270 in the last six years? I mean, these are all people and I can sit down and name them all right now, people I knew.

Raoul Thomas I've lost so many friends. I only have two up (on a bulletin board) right now but at any given point I have at least three, or five articles up about friends who have died. This was about Roger, one of my best friends. This was my boyfriend Bob. I try to keep track but to have it around you, all the time, this whole city would be one great memorial if everybody really faced it. We live the whole AIDS epidemic here. Grief has become an ongoing thing for me. You become numb. Sometimes you just feel like you can't go to another memorial. Some people had really complete deaths. The timing left a completeness to their lives. For others, it's an unfinished book with chapters complete. Some died without saying goodbye to the people they wanted to say goodbye to. I wish we weren't talking about it. Ten years ago, it would have been unfathomable for us, at our age, to be sitting talking about extreme losses of friends. They were all too young.

Re-entry

Peter Groubert After five years of waiting to die, I decided to go back to work and a friend got sick. He worked on an ocean liner in San Diego and was very ill. He had AIDS and didn't know what to do. They got him in touch with a guy who was going to let him be a roommate but the guy wanted sex for putting him up. So I said, "Well that's fucking ridiculous. Get on the plane, come stay with me."

That was 1985 when I first did anything with this room. For the first three years, this room was basically empty. When I knew that Tim was coming, I bought a couch with a convertible sofa, a TV, a stereo. He lived in here for several months during which time, I got involved volunteering on Ward 5A at General Hospital. When Tim got sick and went in, I had a volunteer pass so I could come anytime.

In the meantime, I had also started a group at Davies. They didn't have one so I used the techniques that I learned at Ward 5A, set it up here which helps. After Tim died, I couldn't do any more volunteering. Every room I went into, I saw his face and it just tore me up. What started as a two- or three-hour commitment once a week turned out to be seven days a week at hospital. I got so involved with their lives, their parents, their lovers. After Tim died, it all came to a stop.

New Year in the season of death

Dan Vojir With HIV, I've lost two ex-lovers. I've seen three very good friends degenerate, one that I had to call up his parents in New York and tell them to get the hell out here. He had a hell of a life. "Dan, I gotta show you something." He just discovered it, he had called to say, "We gotta talk about this." He found that they had discovered a lesion on his leg and he didn't know that he was HIV-positive. By sheer accident my doctor, Owen, had a spot available. He went in and within five minutes I got a call from my doctor. I said, "Why are you calling me?" And he said, "The lesions have reached into his lungs." And he said, "You'd better call his parents. This is his last time. He's going to be going back into the hospital and that's it." Oh God. So I said, "Bubbles, they want you in the hospital." And he looked at me and he said, "That means I'm never getting out." That was hard for me.

Bob and I went to his house to get his personal effects and called his parents and said, "You don't remember us but . . ." They came out and so did his brother. Very indicative. He was twenty-three years old. Here was Bubbles on the respirator and looking half the person he had been, just paced back and forth, sort of worried but couldn't bring himself to touch him or come into the room. That was hard. Up until the day he died Bubbles was joking. Our friend June came in, they would always have a laugh. He loved firemen (*laughs a sigh*). But when he looked at me and said, "Basically that means I'm never coming out." That's hard.

We had to go to his funeral. By the way it was New Year's Eve. We had had a party the day after Christmas and he was here. He had been joking. Two days afterwards was when I had to take him to the hospital and then like the day after that he's dead. So, it was New Year's Eve and we had to go to his funeral. Now that's hard. We all remembered him, toasted him and said this is it.

On the present

Cleve Jones *My first interview with Jones took place at the Patio Café on Castro and 18th Street. The date, May 22, 1995, was Harvey Milk's birthday. It also happened to fall the day after the previous evening's AIDS Candlelight Vigil, twelve years after "Fighting for Our Lives."* I don't come in the city very often. I was here a little bit early and I walked around. I could tell you a story about every house on this block and they are not pretty stories. It's very hard. You know, a lot of people don't survive it.

The love of my life killed himself last year. He hadn't gotten sick yet but his T-cells dropped and he just really didn't want to see it unfold over and over. It's so inevitable. You know what's going to happen. You know how horrible it's going to be. So he chose to end it and I'm surprised there haven't been more. What is the most amazing thing is that I still have fun. I still fall in love. I still have a great time. I still love life. I spent time with two friends after the memorial. We drank some wine and we smoked some pot and we told stories about the old days and laughed and laughed and laughed. I think that gay people have a spirit and an ability to get through this somehow. I'm proud of the way we have handled this. It's extraordinary that the gay and lesbian movement has advanced during this time of such suffering and death. The people that I thought were the greatest activists of my time, all tremendous, died. They didn't get to get to Congress or the US Senate. The women are doing it.

There's been so many like him [Bobbi Campbell]. I would like so much to be able to survive this and to tell these stories of how incredibly courageous we were. I know we made mistakes, terrible mistakes and I guess you have to say that we failed in so many respects. I think it's amazing what we have achieved. I think that the gay men with AIDS have . . . if the world could see it, I think the world could learn a lot about courage and dignity and what's important and what's not important. I have. My friends all have. Indescribable horror, to continue to live and to continue to fight. It's pretty amazing. Bobbi was a real role model for me and it's one of the reasons why . . . You know Ricardo chose to end his life before he went through the suffering. He died without having experienced a single opportunistic infection. He didn't want to go through that suffering, but I just really believe that that is what life is about. Life is suffering. Life is pain. When I was young I didn't understand that. I don't think I would want to understand it. But it is about suffering and suffering is inevitable and you are required to go through it. If Bobbi could do what he did, when he did, at a time when there was such fear and ignorance and hate. I've seen so many like that. Marvin had been so sick for a year. He died in, I think it was October of '86. He had everything, tumors through his body, terrible pain. There was no hope and yet he continued. I have seen that over and over, people with absence of rational hope refusing to die, enduring incredible pain, just holding on to their last breath.

I consider myself a Quaker and Quakers worship in silence. You can speak at meetings, only if you are moved by God to do so. It's not like Twelve Steps, you know, sharing what happened today. But I've only, in my whole life, I've only spoken at meeting twice and once was after coming back from saying goodbye to Marvin before he died and really understanding why he refused to die until the body wouldn't let him live any more. It was something that had perplexed me when I watched Bobbi Campbell. When I watched Marvin, and all my friends, I would think where did these people get the courage and the strength and the endurance to keep on going? But watching Marvin die, it was very simple. As long as Marvin was alive, Marvin was being loved and loving back. As long as he was breathing, he was receiving and giving love. That really was what kept him going. All of his family was there and all of his friends. He just really did not want to leave us.

I think this whole experience was about this little group of people who were so isolated from the rest of the world and then to find this kind of tragedy. There are a lot of lessons of this experience that go way beyond boundaries of sexuality, way beyond anything about gay people. I hope our whole experience isn't lost. I don't think it will be.

NINE

Fight Like Hell for the Living

"The two most famous quotes in activist folklore are Joe Hill's 'Don't mourn, organize' and Mother Jones's 'Pray for the dead, but fight like hell for the living.' Although the latter makes a nod at acknowledging the dead, both place the emphasis on political action," Michael Bronski wrote about living in a United States with its selective compassion toward the dying. As the inaction of the Reagan era wore on, G'dali Braverman crossed a fundamental Rubicon leading to ACT UP New York (DeParle, 1990). The battle against the health care establishment he would engage in with ACT UP would help all Americans. If AIDS activists had not hung in there screaming, "We're here! We're Queer! And we're sick!" it's hard to imagine the health care debates of the 1990s occurring. Cleve Jones put the era in context.

Cleve Jones   So there was this first big wave and that was followed by a second angrier wave in the late '80s that gave birth to ACT UP, the Names Project, World AIDS Day, sort of grass-roots political or semi-political actions. I think one of the things that's been confusing for many people is that the Gay/Lesbian Movement and the AIDS movement, I don't really think of the AIDS movement as movement. I think of the Gay and Lesbian Movement as a Civil Rights, as a sexual liberation movement and then you have a response to the epidemic and they become intertwined. People have trouble, I think, keeping them separate. Very different people are driving those two. You still have a lot of people like myself who think of ourselves as Gay Liberationists. Now, you also have a majority of people who are in the movement who don't come from that perspective at all and who have come out in the last ten years. And it's odd for me to watch it sometimes.

Beyond Sister Death

Nancy Lemoins   I don't know. You know, I keep reading these things that compare it to like concentration camp survivors except for we're not going to have any survivors. That's what's really the hardest part of all this. I look at people and I go, this person is going to die, this person who's like so alive and so vibrant. But that's where I get into trouble, when I start judging. I have absolutely no understanding of like what is supposed to work or what's right. My conscious and spirituality are really opposing. I feel politically like it's not OK that people are dying at twenty-five but spiritually I say it's just the way it should be. I don't know. At times I'm really more political than spiritual and then I'll turn around and think that doesn't make any sense at all.

"I really have the desire to have a second dog and name him AIDS so when I am walking him I can call, 'AIDS! AIDS! Come here AIDS!'" long-time activist G'dali Braverman of ACT UP Golden Gate joked as we walked his dog, Quincey, through the foggy hills of his Clipper Heights neighborhood in San Francisco for our early morning interview. "But I am afraid my dog would kill AIDS, which would be the closest thing to a cure we would have achieved." I first met G'dali at an ACT UP march in which we spread the ashes of friends on the grounds of the Capital Building in Sacramento. G'dali advised me on how to hold my hands properly if I were to be cuffed; and did it with an understanding gentleness one would not have expected of such a seasoned veteran. It was his hundredth action since the early days with ACT UP New York. G'dali became involved in AIDS activism in 1982 when it was a group of twenty guys with ironing boards and flyers forming an outfit called Gay Men's Health Crisis warning of impending danger. Twelve years later, "AIDS activism is dangerously close to being on its deathbed," G'dali observed after having watched as those "1000 Deaths" from the old placard have become millions worldwide. This chapter features a lengthy segment on G'dali Braverman. The section has not been edited apart like other interviewees' because of the vividness with which he captures the ethos of ACT UP. The following is G'dali's oral history and the history of a movement. We pick up where G'dali struggled with his spouse's death and the world it showed him. G'dali recalled the hospital where his spouse spent his final days.

G'dali Braverman He was on a wing where there were, at any given point, probably eight or nine AIDS patients, all of whom were going to die in short succession. Nobody was ever released. Once you were in the hospital that was it, that was your last stop. People who were released for a few days would inevitably end up back in the hospital with complications. So, I came to know all these other people who died, before he expired, during their time and their families, you know, started getting familiar with the whole disease on a whole other level.

It completely altered my life. I had never personally dealt with death. I had no idea what a dying person would be like, look like, sound like, you know, kiss like. I had never grieved for that type of a loss or really ever lost. I removed myself from society because I was so devastated by this loss and by the lack of overall support in the world. I really endured that with only one of his friends as a support. I keep saying life was never the same again and it wasn't. I still consider myself a fortunate person. In a way, my life is so charmed that having this happen was that much more of a wake-up call.

Dumped him, picked up ACT UP

I think the root of AIDS activism necessitated our looking at issues around basic gay homophobia to begin to identify why the world wasn't facing up to AIDS. We were not an organized community. We were invisible. We were narcissistic. We pursued our basic primal needs without really thinking, "What is the future direction of our community politically, locally, state-wide, nationally?" You have, basically, masses of people who are closeted or hiding who aren't going to identify themselves under almost any circumstance and accept that risk, even when they are dying. They didn't want to have to deal with the phobias around their sexuality or lifestyle. There was a negative support structure for creating a working environment around the disease.

I met a guy in '87. We were in a relationship for the better part of '87, '88. I had received a couple of flyers in the mail about ACT UP. I breezed through them and, basically, tossed them. I was feeling that I was in this relationship with a generally vacuous person who really didn't seem to have any great concern for the world around him besides how good he looked and which club he was going to. When ACT UP passed we stood on the sidewalk, at Gay Pride in 1988, a year after its formation, I took one look and said, "I am going to go to the next meeting of that organization." There was a sense of power, a sense of action. It didn't appear to be about pity or shame or sadness or guilt. It seemed to be about anger and action. I think that as the individual that I am and as a Jew those were things that I could identify with. So I dumped him, picked up ACT UP.

My first meeting was right after Gay Pride. It was on the first floor and it was packed. People flooded out the doors. People were in the hallways. There was no ventilation. But there was the sense that this was the place to be, all the energy, all the focus around HIV was happening in that room. And I just listened. It was probably young gay men mostly, twenty-three to thirty-five, physically fit, an exceptionally large number of attractive people, energetic, articulate people. Probably 30 to 40 percent of the organization was composed of Jews. Jews have always been at the center of leftist movements which have always ended up fucking them over in the end. An agenda was put together. The meeting went on for three and half hours and people stayed. All ages, sixteen to sixty, the whole gamut. Men, women, boys, girls, parents, but mostly gay men and you didn't know who was HIV-positive or not.

Even from that early time there were only a few of us who identified as positive. I was one of those people. I found out in early '87. I don't remember it definitely. By that time I had accepted the fact that chances were that everybody I knew was going to die and that I was going to die and it was just a question of time. It just seemed the logical conclusion. In retrospect it *was*.

Actions were proposed every week at that point. I can remember feeling a buzz in those earlier demonstrations. I'd be leaving my office or my apartment and walking or being on a subway and having this sense of the unknown in my gut, this feeling that I was putting myself at risk and this response circulating through my blood of "You have to! You must. This is just something that you are going to do" and hearing myself think, "What's going to happen? Is there going to be brutality? Are people going to be fighting? Is there going to be a confrontation? What is my response going to be? Am I going to be able to stick to our non-violent guidelines? Am I not going to feel a need to reciprocate aggression on a physical level?" As a new person you go through this constant inner checks and balances because you are so filled with a fury. We helped perpetuate that anger in the discussions that we had around the actions so that you are a bottle of emotions with a great sense of purpose. When you were at the demonstration you sustained yourself on an adrenaline rush because you were chanting the whole time whether it was a half an hour or an hour and a half. Physically maintaining that energy level does incredible things to you. You walk away from the demonstration feeling elated, really elated and purposeful. I don't think that I ever experienced an overwhelming fear. I always had a sense that I have a good head on my shoulders and that I would know how to respond and react in critical situations.

I, early on, chose to be visible in my work and to take a sort of leadership role in my work as an AIDS activist. I still didn't socialize with AIDS activists, didn't sleep with AIDS activists, didn't seek to establish friendships, and didn't seek out media interviews, but I sought to be central on issues that I chose to work on.

Housing, treatment, and city issues

ACT UP was working on a multitude of issues. There were probably a good twenty committees existing, treatment issues, housing, local issues, city issues, a media committee, etc. There were people working on those issues that were meeting several times a week outside of the regular Monday meeting.

I chose to work on housing for general reasons that it would be difficult to muster people to work on an issue that wasn't a glamorous issue. The committee had just been formed the previous week. The issues the floor was responsive to at that point were local issues and treatment issues around the FDA and the NIH. Housing would be difficult because here we were predominantly middle-class to affluent gay men whose self-perception would be that one would probably never have to deal with becoming destitute and therefore this seemed like a peripheral issue. We would be advocating for mostly a minority population. I thought it would be a challenge to get these organizations to deal with their issues. We turned out to be a very successful committee and mustered large attendance at our demonstrations.

The first demonstration that I was involved with was at the Trump Tower on Fifth Avenue targeting Trump and the City for the millions of dollars in tax rebates that developers like him were receiving. We felt these funds should be going towards low-income housing and the abolition of shelters as primary housing for homeless people and inappropriate housing for homeless people with life-threatening illnesses. We moved on to having several successful demonstrations against the city's Housing Preservation and Development and Housing Works departments. They were very successful demonstrations, in terms of the media pull and getting the public officials to the table to negotiate, and in terms of getting any community response around issues. I think we really were instrumental in the early work that transcended the issues around being a gay man with HIV. After I left New York to come here the committee actually went on to develop an organization called Housing Works which provides housing.

ACTION!!! – The anatomy of a demonstration

I would have to say that one of the most successful demonstrations i
New York proper would have been in 1989, the anniversary action whe
we shut down part of downtown and had a march to City Hall. W
started very early, probably 7:30 in the morning. I recall well over 250
people with a massive picket and incredible posters and propaganda.

On the day of the march there's a sense that there is going to be mas
hysteria, like complete lack of control and organization. That rarel
happened, though. There would be individuals who had volunteered t
be marshals to watch the police interaction with the actual picket lin
There were people who were identified to be media liaisons to identif
media and bring them over to spokespeople to actually address the issue
There were people doing propaganda and people doing just leg
observation and watching the actual arrest procedures and identifyin
police by badge numbers. They would have lists of the people who wer
risking arrest so that nobody would get lost in the system. There wer
lawyers on site. Then there were the separate affinity groups. So you ha
this multifaceted demonstration and everything was happenin
simultaneously. Incredibly, there was a sense of coordination. Rarely di
anything horribly unpredictable happen. Incidents would happen, but i
wasn't as if it overrode the demonstration or resulted in everyone bein
at some heightened risk.

That day the group that I was with decided to take over the street an
block all traffic. It was one of the major streets near City Hall downtow
I think? My sense of geography is pretty bad. So we waited for th
appropriate moment and chained ourselves together and went into th
street and lay down. Then the police went through the crowd of peopl
who were risking arrest. It was rush hour. The last of us probably weren'
arrested until around lunchtime. Then, of course, we would be carted of
in paddy wagons and held. There were probably a couple of hundred tha
were arrested at that demonstration. They weren't able to move u
through the system rapidly enough and they didn't have enough jail spac
to put us through. That was a massive demonstration. It really impacte
both the organization and the city in terms of visibility of the issues.

Those local actions really served to alert people in masses. Th
following week you would suddenly have 800 people at the meetin
instead of 400. It also began drawing media attention and the attentio
of other AIDS organizations to better identifying what was truly goin
on in the system. City bureaucracies were starting to unravel the kind o

corruption within the administrations – that programs like shelters weren't working or that hospitals were overcrowded or that health care was insufficient. Those things that seemed like such highbrow intellectual garble when we started talking about them became commonplace ideas among the mass media.

We went up to Albany, to the state capital. This was like at the 1990 anniversary action. We felt that Cuomo had not been addressing issues on the state level around AIDS, discrimination legislation, and all sorts of stuff. There were fifteen affinity groups there. My housing committee called ourselves the "Mario Antoinettes," targeting Mario Cuomo, and we made or had incredible costumes like Marie Antoinette, big dresses with ruffles and we had wigs. We were in full drag and we carried coffee cake; we went around the state capital in drag screaming, "Mario Cuomo's policy is Let Them Eat Cake!" We went to his office and threw crumb cake around the door. It got wild media attention and it was fun and was poignant and it was hell getting arrested (*sounding campy*) in huge, huge garb. But we did fun things like that. A lot of it was about creativity and attracting the media in new ways and using innovation and art and yet never losing sight of the urgency of AIDS and being able to find new ways to talk about AIDS.

Cuomo's 1990 State of the State

Among the most critical of actions for me was a demonstration two months before that. It was January of 1990, only four months before I moved to San Francisco. There was a group of fifteen of us who were targeting Mario Cuomo and the state legislature around the state budget for AIDS and the lack of response. Mario Cuomo was going to be addressing the state legislature as "The State of the State Address."

We decided we were going to get into the chamber at the state capital and disrupt him. We thought we were going to be able to get passes through an inside source. Basically, it was for elected officials and media and wealthy people. As it turned out, I got in partially out of luck but more out of wit. I put together a bogus story. There were three of us and we were all very well dressed and very presentable and we quickly went up to the entryway. There was a metal detector and they said, "Can we have your tickets?" I immediately separated myself and pretended I wasn't with the other two. We were standing all of six inches away from each other. It was about an hour before he was going to be addressing the chamber. So there were maybe twenty people in the whole chamber in this huge hall and I said, "Well, actually, I don't have my ticket but Senator, I don't know, Willmayer has my ticket. I think that he's in there." And they said, "Well, you can go in and look for him but come right back out if he's not there and you will have to wait back here for the ticket." I said, "Sure, no problem I will be right back in a couple of minutes," knowing that a crowd was gathering behind me and that the security guards were going to forget that I had gone in.

I entered the chamber and went to the farthest point in the room away from the entrance. There was a woman sitting by herself there, middle-aged conservative-looking woman, and I sat two seats away from her. She was reading a newspaper. When I entered the chamber, I identified her and I waved so the security guards would see me and think that I knew someone in there. And I sat next to her and I spent the next half an hour lip-synching, pretending that I was talking to her, but she didn't notice me 'cause I didn't sit directly next to her, but for anyone who was watching me from a distance it appeared as though I was with her. The chamber became more crowded, I maintained my position and I had no idea whether anyone else had gotten in.

I suspected I was on my own, but the agreement that we had made, if we had gotten in in groups, was that at the moment that he said AIDS that would be the moment that we would interrupt him. I knew he was going to say AIDS but I didn't knew where it was going to fall into the speech. My heart was racing and he finally got to the part where he said AIDS and paused first, only for an instant, waiting to see if anyone else would stand up and there was no one and I began screaming about what the state budget was and the inadequacy of his response and the chamber went silent and the cameras all turned to me and him.

His response was brilliant. I made sure I was as far away from both the entrance and the exit so that I would have the maximum amount of time to speak, and as they were coming towards me, people started screaming. He said, "Let the man speak." So I spoke and, of course, he interrupted me. It was something to the effect of lip service but it was well orchestrated lip service and then I retorted. It was clear to him that I wasn't simply going to leave. I was going to debate him and he would leave his platform. So at that point he let them take me out and they literally dragged me through the state chamber.

It ended up on the cover of the New York Times on probably like January the 5th, 1990. There was an article starting with: "Mario Cuomo's State of the State Address," or "Cuomo Gets Heckled." That was probably the riskiest feeling I've ever had.

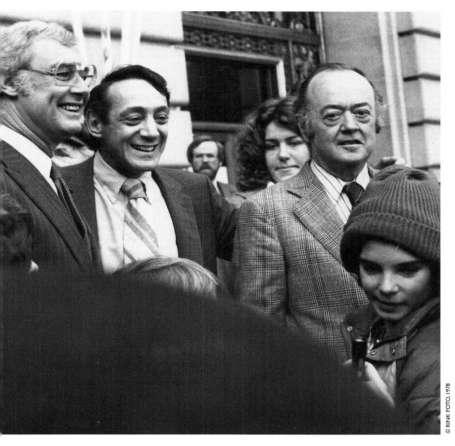

January 1978. Inauguration of
Harvey Milk (second left) with
Mayor George Moscone (left) at
San Francisco City Hall.
Assassinated November 27, 1978.

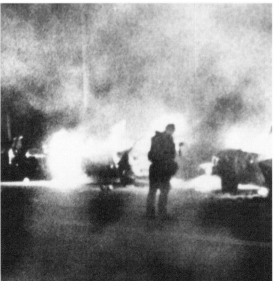

May 21, 1979. "White Night Riot"
at San Francisco City Hall, fuelled
by the sentencing of Dan White
to just seven years'
imprisonment for the murder of
Harvey Milk and
George Moscone.

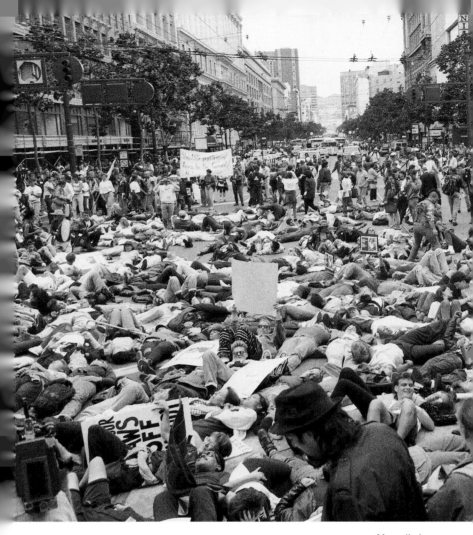

Mass die-in,
San Francisco 1990.

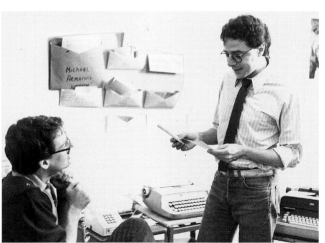

KS office with just two
employees – Cleve
Jones (right) and
Donald Currie.

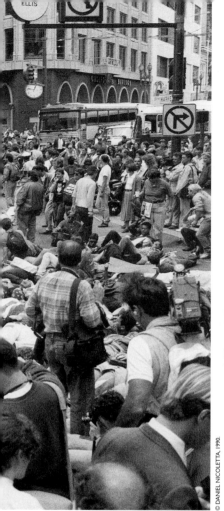

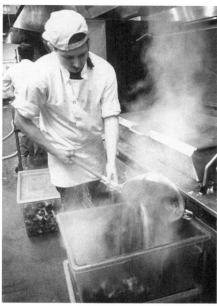

Project Open Hand, San Francisco 1991. A volunteer food program for PWAs.

"Women Get AIDS Too", San Francisco AIDS conference 1990.

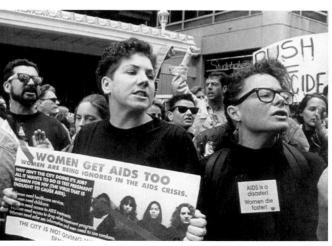

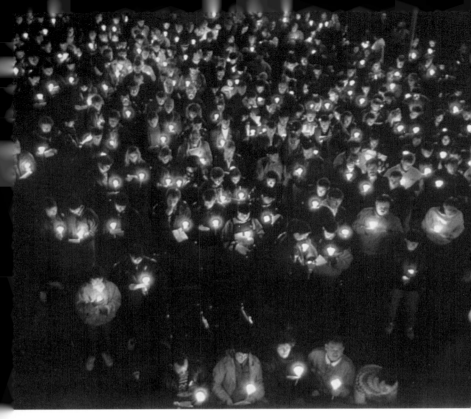

Candlelight vigil, Toronto 1990.

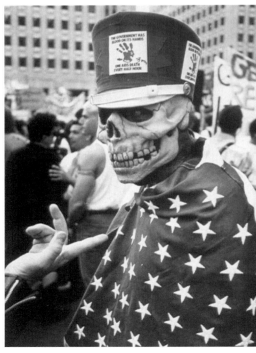

Death flag, San Francisco AIDS
conference 1990.

Brad Sherbert   My circle of friends keeps changing 'cause people die. I don't know what keeps me here so long; I see people doing everything they can to take as much care of their body as possible and they still die very fast. I can remember and I go to the funeral and I just go on. It wasn't too long ago when I used to get real nervous in front of a crowd of people to give a eulogy. Hell, I've had so much practice at it now, I oughta have one gigantic eulogy speech for everybody and just fill in the name (*laughs*). It doesn't make me nervous or anything anymore. It's really hard too. You don't really get used to it but you become accustomed to it. It's the worst thing, I think this epidemic, that anybody could imagine.

Of course I went with ACT UP to City Hall. And we spent the whole day in City Hall raising hell. I got there at ten in the morning and finally at four in the afternoon I got arrested. We didn't know at what time the city supervisors were going to meet. We were going to stay there until we got arrested or they met. Finally they met and, it's like, I sat up and started screaming about the budget cuts and people dying. I told them, "This disease is killing me." And I said, "If you don't allocate money here, here and here, I'm gonna die sooner than I have to." And the one supervisor, I forget her name, Angela Allioto, she's supposed to be our friend. She's like, "Sir, if you'll just take a seat and be quiet, you'll get your turn to speak." And I'm like, "Look, I've been here all day and you're here. That'll affect, how long I will live depends on how much money you allocate and you're telling me to sit down and shut up." I said, "Hell no, I'm not going to sit down and shut up." I kept right on talking and she motioned to the cops, OK come get him.

They put the little plastic handcuffs on me. And, of course, it didn't hurt, they put them fairly loose and stuff and I like kicked and yelled that they were hurting me and screamed (*laughs*). I did not go easily. That's because, if you go peaceably, you don't draw any attention. Well they carted this guy off to jail – but if you make a scene? That night I was on every channel. I was on the front page of the *Chronicle* paper, the front page of the *Bay Area Reporter*. That's what happens when you throw a fit when you get arrested. You go peacefully, they don't even mention it on the news. (*Sardonically.*) The news media reported it as a slightly noisy demonstration (*laughs*). I bet nobody got any work done at City Hall that day, OK.

I'm surprised they didn't arrest me sooner. We had the city supervisors' office blocked off at one point. And it was like, one guy came and said, "I just want to come and get a few of these papers." And I said, "You know what I think of these papers." There was like a stack about two feet tall of all these different forms. I grabbed the whole stack. Took it out of the supervisors' main office, went out to the balcony inside City Hall and just tossed the shit as hard as I could. And I said, "That's what I think about all this red tape bullshit!" I thought for sure I was going to jail when I did that. I thought, God this is too wild to pull this shit and get away with it, you know.

Arrest, core philosophy and the police

G'dali Braverman   There's a point when there's a demonstration where my mother will call me from New York and if I pick up the phone she will say, "I can't believe you are out of jail already. I thought I'd, you know, would leave a message on your voice-mail just saying, 'call me when you get home later.'" I'm not blasé about the importance of civil disobedience and the importance of risking arrest to get your message across. It's just part of my responsibility as an activist.

I can honestly say that I didn't become an AIDS activist to save my life. I didn't have that as an ulterior motive. I became an AIDS activist because I felt that the whole system was corrupt and that our government was at fault for the spread of this disease and that we needed to wake up. It was about the world. It really was about the world and about our world as a gay people, which I still recognize and believe will be annihilated because of this epidemic. As our community becomes more passive, more reticent, I can see those AIDS activists who are left saying that old adage, "Help yourself first so you can help others." Many of us are at a mid- to late stage of disease where if we don't survive and there aren't any new people coming into it, then we can't do anything to help future generations. Ultimately that hasn't been my objective. My philosophy is that this epidemic will be with us for at least another generation and therefore we should do everything in our power to keep the urgency of AIDS focused in the public eye.

The crashes

We talked for a few minutes about the emotions around demonstrations – the adrenaline and the post-demo isolation. You're really jostling my memory now and all sorts of fun things are coming out, and the horrible things. When you're in jail, waiting to be released or sighted out, it's a weird feeling because you've suddenly gone from this energy of a crowd and a demonstration and your action that you planned down to the final detail to being a hostage. You can feel very trapped and it can be a very unpleasant, hot, unsanitary, disease-ridden environment to be in. You feel very disempowered. They seek to make you feel that way for the most part. Although I have been in many situations where I felt the police were more than compliant, that they were actually aiding and abetting us in ways which I really respected.

I was arrested in Albany three times. The first time I interrupted Mario Cuomo at the State of the State. And the officer that arrested me, he pulled me out and then headed me over to this big burly officer, 250 pounds. And I turned to him and I said something like, "Just don't mess my hair up." And he looked at me and I winked at him. We both started laughing and we became buddies. When I came back in my Mario Antoinette outfit, he actually sought me out. I mean there were officers all over the State Building following different people and he asked to arrest me so that we could hang out (reveling in the memory). This is an upstate New York middle-aged married guy, you know, and we developed this connection. And that wasn't the last time that happened to me with a police officer. I never hid that from my co-activists, even the ones that are the most dire cop haters. The third time that I came back he asked some other activists that he had arrested, "So where's Braverman?" Someone else arrested me and he came over and said, "Sorry I didn't get you this time, you know." I think several of us have had that kind of a rapport because we didn't turn as we were getting arrested and say, "Fuck You! You God damned Pig!" and spit on the guy. If you can just turn and say, "Hey look, I know you are doing your job. Do me a favor, don't put the cuffs on too tight, I've got bad circulation. I'm a person living with AIDS." Or "Do you know anyone who's died?" I can't tell you how many times an officer has turned to me and said, "My brother died. My brother's sick. Do you have some information?" One time we got arrested here in San Francisco shortly after ACT UP Golden Gate was formed and we were brought into the North Station, and the lieutenant said, "So what phase of clinical trials is this drug in?" If you are always going to assume that the cops are ignorant or that they are on a different side, then you are wrong. You shouldn't and you can't make that assumption. The last time I got arrested, a month and a half ago, the cop said, "You know, my wife has been battling cancer and I'll tell you, the system just fucks people." I don't believe that they're my enemy. I'm not an activist because I have a disrespect for human life. I'm an activist because I respect human life and the need for a quality of life.

But afterwards, when we left a demonstration in the early days we had this sort of unspoken understanding that we would gather, those of us that had been arrested. Or some of us would gather in groups, go get something to eat, or hang out at someone's house, or spend the rest of the day together because of the crash. The emotional crash that comes afterwards is intense because for those instants of the demonstration you forget that you're not living at the tail end of an epidemic. You forget that everything that you are demanding is not going to be achieved when the demonstration is over. You are so focused on the moment that you, somewhere in your mind, believe that the solution is here, in the action and clearly it isn't. This is just part of the process. So when you end up home alone afterwards, you wake up to the fact that death is still here, your friends are still dying, you're still sick, the system still exists as it was and that some changes may come about but it's just the beginning. One of the difficult things of being an activist is maintaining that high level of energy and motivation and not letting the crashes destroy you. My crashes were always short-lived 'cause I was always so busy organizing another project. I think in the earlier days, particularly in New York, there were so many people and there was such camaraderie that it was easy to stay focused and to feel a sense of support. With today's attrition, that doesn't exist.

Dan Vojir The ends are very noble. I used to get upset at ACT UP. I think they've calmed down bit. I think they've done a lot for people. In fact, there was one woman I was talking to. Her child has Down's Syndrome. She's practically reversed the Down's Syndrome in the child by using certain smart drugs. She said, "You know something, if it weren't for ACT UP my kid wouldn't be alive today." I says, "Why?" because her child didn't have HIV. She says because it was ACT UP that got the FDA to accept the mail order drugs that we finally get in the country. She says, "I totally support everything ACT UP ever does because of what they did for my child actually, inadvertently." She says, "A lot of people don't know that ACT UP did a hell of a lot of stuff for a lot of other people who don't have AIDS."

Jay Segal You only do drugs for one reason and that is to stall the progression of the disease until a cure comes along. Realistically, you're not going to see the cure, not for about another forty years, maybe. I've learned a lot about AIDS, joined both groups of ACT UP, got things changed. They're the only people on this planet that have made any changes. Congress wouldn't have changed on its own. The President wouldn't have done anything on his own. I don't always agree with them but they work. This country was built on activism. Look at the Boston Tea Party, talk about a major demo. They took a whole bay. We just trashed ships. And ACT UP is good activism. The cause is good.

I was heavy into ACT UP in Chicago. Dealt with a couple of major demos on health care and alternatives. The Chicago Demo, I was significant in that one in its inception and creation. ACT UP is a bunch of sick sissies who can't agree on anything that somehow get a lot of work done. Strangely enough, in almost every major AIDS conference that's ever going to happen this year, ACT UP is on the committees, ACT UP is on the speakers lists. ACT UP is a reputable source now because they've dealt with it more. They are personally impacted.

Cleve Jones I produced all the candlelight marches for the first eleven years. The tenth anniversary of the murders of Harvey Milk and George Moscone, I woke in the middle of the night, Oh, I know exactly how to do this this year. And I came up with this scenario that I would have a bare stage with a single spot. As we started with candles and I had the stage be totally dark and then without any announcement, a single spotlight, I wanted Joan Baez to walk out on stage and without any other words to sing, "I dreamed I saw Joe Hill last night, alive as you and me, I said Joe you're ten years dead, I never died said he, I never died said he." And I called her up and she said, "Oh, yes, that would be fabulous." And she did it. There's been about a half dozen times in my life where I saw something so clearly and then got to see it just as I'd imagined. She came out. The crowd recognized her before she got to the microphone, but her voice was so distinctive they knew it and there was an electricity through the crowd. It was Joan Baez and she was singing this great labor song that applied to our situation and had this thread of continuity. It was faaaabulous!!!

Inspiration for the Names Project

'85, when I had the idea of the quilt, to give you an idea of the extent of my full arrogance, I organized the Candlelight March, I decided that I wanted it to be a perfect night, therefore I would be the only speaker (*laughing*). We marched on City Hall and in the hours before the march I passed out a stack of cardboard placards and markers. Everybody wrote down one name. And I gave my fabulous speech:

"Now our numbers have been diminished and many among us have already been condemned to an early and painful death. But we are the lesbians and gay men of San Francisco and though we are again surrounded by uncertainty, we are survivors. We will survive again."

But we went to the Federal Building and I had ladders hidden around the shrubbery at the Federal Building. We climbed up three stories and covered the thing. As I was walking through the crowd, I looked at it and I said, "it looks like a quilt" and immediately thought of my grandma and the quilts that have been passed down through our family. Then it was like a slide falling into place. I just saw this massive quilt with the dome of the Capital Building in the background. It was almost two years later that we first unfolded the quilt.

PART IV

Families, Evolving Demographics, and Otherness

TEN

Waves Beyond Borders

AIDS hit regions of the globe in varying degrees and they responded in turn. The reputation of the San Francisco Model of AIDS treatment grew. Border crossings have always been problematic for PWAs. As the plague raged, people from all over the world migrated to survive and heal through access to the San Francisco Model. Interviewees recall the anguish, dilemmas and successes of their journeys from and memories of AIDS in Mexico. Interviewees reflect on the battles to maintain a sense of themselves through the double and triple forms of stigmatization as they make their ways through an American culture that outlaws services to immigrants, barely tolerates homosexuality, and tends to deny the existence of those with disease.

As the grim realities and grotesque treatments he was receiving intensified, Gabriel Martinez moved to San Francisco in search of a little ingenuity in terms of treatment. Gabriel had just moved into our housing program when I began to work there. "Ciao caro," Xico used to greet me. Italian fits the way they looked at things. They both had long hair, great smiles, late nights, Gay Pride parades, and socializing to attend to. Hugo, who lived in the building, took a more serious outlook. Marcos Reyes used to visit to participate in the Positive Art Program. Gab's old boyfriend with whom he moved from Mexico made frequent visits. Santo, a friend from Sacramento, came a lot. Eventually he even moved into the building. His health caught up first.

One morning Gab and Xico arrived with heads shaved right in step with a city in which images of disease overlapped with style. They had just gotten back from the hospital where Santo had gone into chemotherapy and they wanted to put him at ease. Another Sunday Gab, Xico and the rest of the group left in drag, only to return a couple of hours later and change back into jeans before the sun had gone down. I asked Gab why. "For Santo's spirits. We were just visiting him." Santo passed away a few months later. Gab's old boyfriend soon followed. Xico soon began taking more and more trips to the emergency room himself, "Please, don't even get sick . . ." Xico whispered from his doubled-over position, looking up for a moment, as he sat in the lobby waiting for Gab to get the car on one of those trips. Xico is now bedridden.

The day of the interview, short, brown-haired, handsome twenty-eight-year-old Gabriel Martinez wears jeans, hiking boots and a five o'clock shadow. We sit at the living room table of his apartment covered by movie posters and plants overlooking a park and talk about those old friends. Gab grew up with nine sisters and a few more brothers in Mexico. He recalled the first cases of AIDS he heard of in Guadalajara.

Gabriel Martinez There were two cases of AIDS that were reported there. I think it was in 1985 or '86. They were the first two cases of AIDS that were reported there. One of my teachers was working for a county hospital, so that's how he knew about it. My homework was to go and interview one of them and find out as much as I could about them and about the disease. I went to see them but they were separated from the rest of the patients in a special room. They couldn't go in and out of the room.

And there was, of course, not much information and most of it was propaganda; information came through the newspapers, most of them from here in San Francisco or health letters from other places. But there was not any government or city education on AIDS or prevention. Most of it was like: don't have sex or don't have sex with males. The Church has the power to either accept things or not. They do condemn the use of condoms. Talk was between gay people who would get together and make comments, "Oh, I read about this" or "I had a friend who traveled to some other place" and will comment whatever they heard.

And that went on until about 1988, mostly because to take the test you had to give them your name and address. You'd have to give them a list of sexual partners for the last two years and telephone numbers, apparently to contact them and make them aware of taking a test. So it was more like, if you came out positive saying, Well here's this list that you have sex with. Let's test all of them and they will be linking you directly like you infected this many persons. It was very discriminatory, so nobody wanted to take the test. There was no respect or confidentiality at all.

When I started having friends with HIV it was mostly between gay males that they would make comments. Also it was the wrong idea about, "Well, you can tell when somebody has AIDS 'cause they will look like this and that and that," and that was the main misconception too. "Oh well, you look healthy," or "I'm healthy. Look at me." So mostly it was misinformation. In the town, sexual education doesn't really exist. It's mostly dominated by the Church. Five years ago the government was doing some big signs that displayed condoms. Because the Church objected they took down all that propaganda about condoms. They are very reluctant to it. People are using them more, but still.

Testing

It took me almost three years to decide on having a test. I couldn't avoid it any more. In 1988, when I came to California to live here, I had to have taken the blood test. I was in San Fernando. I called them two days later, they say, "Something went wrong with them but we have the same samples so you don't have to come back again. Give us another two or three days." So I gave them another two or three days and then I went to the clinic. One of the nurses, the one who was supposed to take care of me, she saw me, she stepped back one or two steps. She was like really horrorized and called another nurse who took me and then told me I was positive. The first nurse, she didn't want to touch me or have anything to do with me. This was like here in California. I was like, "Wow, oh my God." That gave me an idea. Then the other nurse told me, "Keep going on with your life. There is help here. Get into one of the county hospitals to be tested to see your CD count. And just take it easy, you are not alone."

And I had my partner with me. We had decided to come to the U.S. together. When he got back from work, he asked me how the tests came out and I say, "Fine," but I didn't tell him anything. I was hoping he would come out negative. And so I went with him. There was a very young nurse, like sixteen or seventeen years old, and she gave him the results. He was, of course, shocked. She was the one that was crying instead of my boyfriend. He came out and he told me, "Well, I'm positive," and asked me, "You were suspecting it? Right?" And I said, "Yes." "You knew it?" I say, "Well, yeah I'm positive too." And then he said, "Well you lie to me." "I didn't lie," I say, "Everything was OK by that moment."

It was the first time I was living in with him and away from my family and learning the language and having everything different. Our relationship was fading. The only thing that I did, I went to this small outpatient clinic. They told me, "Oh, I'm sorry. We're not doing anything here. You have to go to L.A. to go and get care and probably some experimental drugs. We don't have any of that here. It is not accessible and we don't have personnel that is trained to do anything."

Then I moved up to Sacramento with some friends and I spent two years there. That's when I sort of started. I went to a county hospital and I got my first CD4 count. I was happy there. I had a lot of friends and I was working. I wasn't feeling very well because for the last six months I was on AZT and my body couldn't tolerate it any more. It was making me sicker when I took it than when I stopped taking it. I talked to my doctor about it and I remember telling him about DDI which was the newest drug. He just said, "No, I cannot give you DDI and you have to keep on AZT. That's the only medicine we're giving to HIV-positive people." He told me, "We are about to increase the dosage from 600 to 1200 per day." And he said, "If you don't want to take it then I'm not going to see you again." So I was feeling really sick and I had a friend who lived here. He was talking to me. He was, "Why don't you move down there and you can move into my place until you get a job and then you can move on your own. There are more options, more treatments and there are better doctors that can treat you nicer. You have a better chance to survive because AZT is going to kill you."

Moving to San Francisco

So I left everything and I moved down here with him. I got into San Francisco General and I started seeing another doctor who put me on DDC. It did work for two months but I didn't really feel I was getting any benefit so I started on DDI and it was the same. I was at least hoping to stabilize so we stopped and he enrolled me into that D4T.

I wasn't very happy here because I left my work and all my friends in Sacramento. I didn't have any friends in the city. When my doctor saw my papers and my CD4 count, he told me, "Sign all those papers and you can just go on disability. You don't have to worry about anything else." And I say, "But I want to work." So I got a job and I went for four months and I was kind of happy even though it was hard to get up in the mornings. *Eventually, health realities slowed the pace and Gabriel quit his job.*

My dwindling circle

In this time that I have been positive so many people that I have known have died, so it is scary. Even if you take good care of yourself something very unpredictable can happen, or you think you are taking good care of yourself and you're not, and you never know, especially living at the building. From all the people that I first saw moving into the building, which was around sixty, only ten of them, I would say five of them are still alive. The rest of them are dead. And people that I used to see doing OK, somehow they would just get stressed out. I guess the biggest problem with this is fear because fear can just kill you. You don't feel like eating. You don't feel like doing anything. You cannot sleep; you cannot rest; you cannot do anything.

And just having the ambulance like every day getting into the place, it used to be even like three or four times a day when the people started getting sick. I used to live on the second floor. It seemed like most of the time they were getting through my apartment into the building and I will hear all the noises. Some days I would just think, "One of these days, it's gonna come and get me. They are going to come and pick me up."

The day I first formally interviewed Hugo, a former Seminary student in his late twenties, he lay in a dark room with pink curtains, yellow dividers, a pump, in a mechanical bed with stainless steel girders in Ward 5D of San Francisco General Hospital. The TV was attached to the wall across from the bed. A Dixie cup, phone, and meds sat on a tray on his bedside table. Hugo's a 5' 5" Latino with brown hair. His parents were from Mexico although he grew up in Texas. He wore wire-rimmed glasses and a white hospital gown with snowflake decorations. Hugo was recovering from a fever as we talked. I tried to ask about the atmosphere but he shut me up, "This ugly room is awful, Benjamin. Being in the hospital is not too exciting." I had known him from the building. The hospital interview was spliced in with previous informal interviews. "This will be the most wonderful year of my life. I can already feel that some wonderful things will unfold this year," Hugo repeats on optimistic days. "Benjamin, I want to ask you a question. Do you know what life is?" he asked from his hospital bed. "I think that life is a sexually transmitted, incurable disease. Just thought I'd tell you that line. I thought it was a good joke." He went on telling about coming to the city and his ins and outs within the San Francisco Model.

Hugo Manzo The very first day I came to San Francisco was very funny. I came to San Francisco on December the 18th of 1990 because I had heard people with HIV are treated better in San Francisco. It was weird because I had stolen this one ticket from El Paso to San Francisco from my cousin. The only things I had with me were a carton of cigarettes, my coat, a little clothes that I had and three dollars. I didn't know what to do so I asked for directions for a Salvation Army. I stepped in San Francisco at one o'clock that day and I walked till about ten o'clock that night looking for a shelter. Finally, at ten o'clock I found a shelter.

I stayed at that shelter for a couple of days. After two days in San Francisco I decided to stop into the San Francisco AIDS Foundation to get information or to decide which way they could help me and luckily they moved me to another shelter. They secured me a bed for thirty days at the AIDS Foundation Emergency Housing. I ended up staying for four months. By that time I had already became a volunteer. Then I moved to one of the Shanti Houses and I lived there for a year which was a bad experience because other people that were living there were drug addicts. I began using drugs, cocaine. I said to myself, I have to move, so I asked my Shanti House Coordinator to move me out of that house and he put me in another house and I stopped doing drugs. I moved out of that house and my life became my life again.

Marcos Reyes *The trip from the Mexico City of his youth through testing positive and moving to a country where Mexicans are assumed to be laborers did, however, provide its share of anguish for Marcos Reyes, a man with a university degree. The fact that he was also gay and positive didn't make things any easier.* It never occurred to me I was going to be up here in the States. My idea was to go to Europe and how did I end up here I swear I don't know. But one day I said, I have to do something in order to have the adventure that I was going for. I sold everything. I got rid of everything and I said, "OK, I am ready for whatever," and L.A. was my destiny at that time. Why L.A.? I guess I knew somebody there. HIV wasn't in my plans. Like two weeks before I was planning on coming, my partner asked me to get tested with him. I wasn't scared or concerned because from the little stuff that I knew, it was you have to be promiscuous, blah, blah and all that moral kind of stuff. This was one day before when I had to get my results, one day before I had my ticket. So it was like a combination of things. I was getting rid of everything and suddenly I got these results and it was like, Ah, oh no (*breaths in and out deeply*) – limbo for a little while, disconnected. I couldn't understand emotionally. I heard they told me that my results were positive and suddenly I felt like I was trapped in a glass. You know when you have a blurry vision that you can't see very well. The results on my partner were negative so I couldn't understand that situation because we were monogamous.

Then I call up at that time and I told him. He was the first person that I disclose my HIV status to after my diagnosis. So that is how it happened.

No counseling, nothing, it was '87, Mexico City, they didn't know any better. So I thought I was going to die for sure in two years or even less, but when did I contract the virus? It has to be at least four years before when I got my results. So according to my logic, it had to be like around '81 when I was infected.

On one side, I thought that I was going to be killed in Mexico City. Being gay was not very socially accepted. Now, you're HIV-positive, that's a fear that you have to face. So I was very scared. I had many plans to do something great out of my life. The other part was that I was always thinking that people was going to be able to look at my face and find out that I was HIV-positive. It was all this deal about secrecy. You don't tell anyone. You keep this for yourself.

The next day I took the bus, by the way, two days from Mexico City to L.A. And I remember that trip because in some ways, it was like a new chapter of my life. It was the very first time I was going away from the city by myself. I didn't know what I was going to do. I said I didn't know anyone. I didn't speak the language, you name it. That was a contradiction about being scared and thinking about death like a relief. I remember one scene coming up here on the bus. We were, I guess, crossing Senora. It was like one day in the desert and nothing else but dunes and dunes. It was a very empty place and that was like how I felt about my life in that moment. I didn't know exactly what I was.

Once in the US, I was living with this family in L.A., a Hispanic, a Latino family. I had been in psychoanalysis in Mexico City and kept up with my therapist. Somehow one of the letters about my status got lost and the family that I was living with found it and asked me to go away from them. That was one of the first encounters I had with rejection.

I was in Los Angeles two months working as a bus boy. That was a cultural shock and then I took the test again. So that was another thing because I didn't know where to go or how to use the services or where to go but I did it. To my surprise it came out positive again as well. I guess I'm positive, you know. At that time I was really trying to understand where I was going. For a couple of years I traveled back and forth between Mexico and here. Finally I decided I was going to stay here. One of the reasons is that the gay movement was stronger up here as well as the AIDS activities. There were more organizations around the subject. I thought, if I want to save my life, I had to do something. At that moment it was the only answer that I had, the only option that I kind of see in my future. So I decide to stay.

I decided San Francisco for the change of life again, new adventures probably. My life was getting, at that stage, very flat. I had a good job, I was a manager at a pet supply store. It was a good job in some senses and a really bad one in some others. I had always been a very highly motivated person. I was doing many things at once. I was volunteering, I had a full-time job, go to school, so I was very busy. By that time, we are talking about one year, a year ago, I was too tired in my full-time job and I guess my immune system wasn't working as well as before. I was getting all these physical complications out of stress and I was ready to try something new again. A friend of mine said to me he wanted to move up here and I said, "OK, lets go to San Francisco and see how it works." And I like it, it's a little city. I like that. I like the political involvement that people have up here. It is motivating. It seems like you have a voice so I like that.

ELEVEN

HIV, Family, and the Other

The spectrum of HIV highlights many of the previously existing dimensions of class, race and gender biases existing in American culture (McKenzie, 1991). From the onset of the epidemic, HIV high-risk groups (gays, minority status women, intravenous drug users (IVDUs)) have lived within margins categorized as less than 100 percent American, as "the other," by the dominant culture (Heale, 1990). As late as 1995, Jesse Helms was still analyzing the problem by pointing out, "People get it by engaging in self-destructive, disgusting behavior" (Jacobs, 1995). Helms might as well have come out and called PWAs diseased pariahs, if he hasn't already. The attitude has trickled down to the masses. For those who think these attitudes don't have an influence, tell that to Pat and Fred Grimes, two PWAs, whose mailman failed to deliver their mail for weeks because he was afraid of contracting the AIDS virus from their mail (AP Wire Service, 1995). Stories such as these abound.

Neglect is perhaps the most profound form of abuse. In response to the epidemic, Reagan didn't utter the word AIDS in public until 1986, much less lead the country to take on the epidemic. By its silence the Federal Government delivers the message that people with AIDS as "the other" are expendable. Today, according to the CDC, AIDS is the number one cause of death for all men and women between twenty-five and forty-four, yet PWAs are still considered "the other" (Weir, 1995).

HIV and the American family

The role of the family within the AIDS pandemic cannot be underestimated. A central question of life with HIV concerns how one will die: alone or with a family? People follow several routes: some go home to die with their birth families or with members of an extended family; others depend on anonymous health-care workers in a hospital or hospice; and others die by themselves. Unfortunately, a huge number are rejected by their families because they have a disease that families, for reasons of ignorance and prejudice, perceive to be different from other diseases. Women have twice the burden, because they have not only their own lives to worry about, but those of their offspring.

The following chapter examines the vexing question of the relationship of "the other" to the American family. Central questions around American attitudes toward deviance lie at the root of such themes as: How does "the other" fit into the American family? Do American families create their "others"? Will the American family accept "the other" or engage in a case of conditional love by rejecting/neglecting family members with HIV?

Marija Mrdjenovic Major illness in the past has been described as "their problem." Syphilis, for example, was always seen as the "French disease" by the British, and the "British disease" by the French, because they hated each other. Other illnesses, such as the bubonic plague, were seen as condemnations by God, when in fact, they were just something as simple as having killed off too many cats who were keeping the rat populations under control (Shepard, 1995).

John Cailleau Being gay, prior to the '70s, was an incredibly unpopular thing to be. The attachment of AIDS to a group of people who were incredibly unpopular to begin with, against whom there was plenty of overt and covert discrimination, added up to a mysterious, transmittable disease carried by this group of "horrible" people. You end up with that do-nothing situation that Randy Shilts wrote about for so many years.

Richard Chavez I think we've lost a little bit in terms of what we want in this country. This country has a consciousness and has a personality as a whole. It also has a shadow side to it which it raises every so often through the century as it grows older. The shadow decisions are coming closer and closer together as we mature as a civilization. We're letting that make our decisions for us.

There's "us" and "them": always, "we're not them." "It's not us; it's the other ones . . ." That's part of it, part of the blackness . . . You know, gay, it's "them." It's "their" disease. We can't get it because it's something that they do, kind of thing. And it's an, "Oh well, they're not normal anyway. They've got an extra brain cell or something." Whatever the thinking is. That's where the dragging of the feet came in because of the unimportance of our lives, period. These differences which used to be why everybody wanted to be in this country. We're different and well, you know they do things and that's their disease. You can only get it from them. You can't get it from them because you're not gay. I think they forgot that the disease was a human thing and not a lifestyle thing.

Ronnie Ashley *He comments about the factors involved with why PWAs have been treated like they have during the first generation.* Ignorance, hatred, stupidity, racism, sexism, classism, all of it. We always act on our fear, on our ugliness before we think and research and look. Instead of embracing our community, we shoot our community. We separate our community into those who will have and those who will have not, on an economic level, on a cultural level, on a moral level, on a religious level all the way across the board. That's very ugly but just like the genocide of my own people (*Native Americans*), that was done out of fear, ignorance, racism, hatred. All the atrocities are all under the same crap.

Robert Boulanget His [Phillip's] mother was one of those who was afraid of the Russians and I said the Russian people are nice people. They look like you and me and they are blond and brunettes. I saw the people and I didn't see the government. She says, "Well you move there if . . .," you know. She hadn't travelled very much. She wasn't comfortable with other people. We spent Mother's Day, Easter, Thanksgiving and Christmas with her. Whenever I was there she always wanted to be alone with Phillip.

HIV, sex, and the family

Paul Greenbaum Coming out was a big issue, discussing it with my family. But I never sought anyone's approval or acceptance. Basically, I think my other sister, Dot, is uncomfortable with the whole issue of gay life, AIDS, and I might go as far as to say sex in general. But everyone defines, you know, the religious right uses the word homosexual, not gay. The "homosexual activist" and the "homosexual agenda" because the "sexual" is the thing that sticks in people's throats. Why am I any more sexual than my heterosexual niece? I don't refer to her as being heterosexual, although that's fine, but I don't emphasize the sexual issue when describing her. I just sleep with somebody different; sexuality is not all that I am. Everything that I do isn't with a sexual overtone any more than it is with your straight co-workers. In other words, anything that pertains to sex gets a lot of people upset.

Hazel Betsey *A short African-American woman, she wore shorts, glasses and combat boots and explained to me how family dynamics played a key role in her evolution and eventual decision to move to California.* I didn't come here until 1986. I was basically home with my family. I have stepbrothers, the youngest of nine children. So I was in an interesting spot, well protected, more than I wanted to be but then not in a lot of ways too.

I was raised a Jehovah's Witness, was baptized when I was thirteen, and I was active in that until 1981. My Dad was thrown out of the house at that time. He fooled around a lot, was an alcoholic. So it was just me and the boys and Mom. Mom got involved with that religion when I was three. When I was twenty-one I decided I didn't want religion any more. I got into a relationship with a woman there. Before that, I should say I (*laughs*) had boyfriends throughout my life.

I was a victim of incest, I want to say that, throughout my life, various family members. OK, so that was kind of messed up but it didn't hit me hard until I got in my early twenties, like twenty-one it really started to mess with me. That's why I say I wasn't getting the protection that I should have gotten as a little girl in that family. So around that time it really started fucking with me, I said I gotta get away from here. The religion wasn't protecting me. Nothing was protecting me, God wasn't. So that's how I got in a relationship with a woman, a very abusive relationship. I was with her for a few years.

I was really heartbroken over this relationship. Infidelity got involved. It just broke my heart that she would do that. I thought, I gotta get away. I couldn't be there because of my family, because of my friends in the religion. When I left the church, I was thrown out, actually. Disfellowship is what they call it. So I wasn't able to associate with any of my past friends and my family either. I was really ostracized, so I decided that I wanted to get out of the state of Connecticut. I wanted to go somewhere far.

Art *He recalls the meeting with his father in '82 both to come out and to tell him about his new health status. Even though his father was British, the story still illustrates a painful American incapacity to face up to sex, even when the lives of American children are on the line.* My mother was fine; she was fairly willing to discuss the important things that have to be discussed. My father on the other hand, he found out in the same day that not only was I not well but that I had been sleeping with men. He was in Chicago and we met in a hotel in New York. We talked for most of the afternoon and never once mentioned gay. We walked around it. It was this situation and what could happen and we never addressed the sexuality issue at all. Nothing, and I actually got off on it. It took me a year to realize what a horrifying situation it was. He's British and you just don't talk about certain things. I didn't think it was appalling. Hah! (*Chuckles.*) Looking back now, I realize what a shutdown that time must have been to think that that was OK.

Hugo Manzo I was having financial problems so I called home to ask for money, a one-shot deal. After three months I received a check for $40 which was not even enough to cover the phone bills from calling home. So I wrote my mother a letter and I told her that I felt like she would never accept me because of my homosexuality. She wrote back telling me that she could not understand how God would condone the homosexual lifestyle. I gave her the last seven years of letters and calls to know me and she has blown it. They didn't write me or call on Christmas. My family just doesn't get that I am going to die soon. A year ago, I could not even conceive of the thought of dying without my mother by my side but now I can face it. I can see that I will be OK.

Family dynamics with the other

Cynora Jones I come from a business family. My baby sister is on Wall Street; she's pretty much accepted that I have this. Recently the minister of her church disclosed he's HIV-positive. (*Whispers.*) She doesn't understand it. (*Screams.*) She understands it with me but she doesn't understand that her pastor has just come out! You see what I'm saying? "I can see how that might have happened to you," and she's got a master's. It's irrational thinking that goes along with this disease. "God got you." See, I could see that happening. "You knew you weren't supposed to do that. You're not gonna get away with that." The way I break through the stigma is more people like myself. More people like me need to come out and say, "I have it. Fuck you, if you don't like it."

Marija Mrdjenovic grew up in Independence, Missouri. Her family had fled from Yugoslavia, where she was born, because of pressure from Tito. That was the '50s. US Government officials kept a close eye on them to make sure they were not perpetrating any sort of un-American activities, nothing subversive. After graduating from Brandeis, Marija moved to San Francisco in 1979 to follow her calling.

She has sandy blond hair, vivid eyes and a body losing strength. Although she accredits her HIV status to a blood transfusion, Marija never branded herself an "innocent victim" as Kimberly Bergalis did in blaming her dentist for her status (Applebome, 1990).

Marija Mrdjenovic In August of '82 I went to a beach party out at Drake's Bay with the people from the Renaissance Faire where I was working. After the party, my boss was driving and we had an accident. I had to be taken to the emergency room at Novato Community Hospital where I was given two units of packed red blood cells where I was probably infected.

When I tested positively, I couldn't help but think back to that accident and the blood transfusion. Although there was a really good likelihood, my boyfriend was not infected. It was a shocker to me. I said to him, "I know that we have been seeing each other for a while, and I have no idea how much time I have but if you'd like to get married, I'd like to get married." And so he said, "Yeah, sure, let's get married." We went back to New York and met his family. They all seemed very nice towards me and very friendly. I'd met with the reverend, and we didn't seem to have any problems with the marriage, no questions, no nothing. Afterwards we walked across the street to this park and that's where his sister told me that the wedding was off. He was sitting there but he didn't have the courage to tell me himself. I was obviously devastated but I was also very angry, and I swore to them at that time that I would survive this, just to prove them wrong. When we came back out here, he packed up all of his things and left for Los Angeles without really talking to me. I asked him to please not contact me again because it would be much easier for me to just have him gone like he has died or something. So I was then alone out here.

His sister definitely had a problem with AIDS. I think that she was afraid that I was going to be too much trouble for him and I was using her little brother. She also was very devout and wanted to make sure his first marriage would be his last. I think that may have figured into the thing. Why marry this girl if she's just going to die? You know?

For nine months, I was pretty much alone. I figured that I was just not going to meet anyone; I was just going to live as best I could. Then, in the fall of '88, I started doing a show again. It was a Christmas show at Dickens Faire here at Pier 45½, same as the Renaissance Faire folks. I was asked to do a comedy spoof of a Dickens family story. My son was a man named Mitch. For some reason he started to take an interest in me. I thought, "That's all very well and good, but nothing's going to come of it, and he's a very sweet, good-looking man. As soon as he knows about my health, that's going to be the end of it." We would talk and go for coffee and things like that. Finally one night it got very very romantic and I had to tell him. That was the hardest thing in the world that I've ever had to do – the hardest. Finally I got it out and he said, "Well, couldn't we use condoms?" (*Laughs.*) I realized, yes, yes we could. He moved in two months later. We married two years ago, on Valentine's Day. It was very charming. He's been with me, supporting me, and doing partners studies with me. He is why I am alive. I know there are a lot of people out there who don't get that kind of support; they, generally speaking, get abandoned by their family and friends.

At first my mother was so shocked, she said, "Yah, vhy did you ever go to San Francisco?" She's German, obviously. She was angry that I'd gone because maybe I wouldn't be infected if I'd stayed back in Missouri away from all the crazies in San Francisco. But once she began to realize exactly what was going on, that this was my health and I had to fight it, she became the best coach a person can have; she is always on the lookout for anything that might help. But then, during WW II she and her family were forced out of their home by the Russians, and she had to care for her mother, her father and her sister, all of whom died of different types of TB. She slept with them, and she never got it because she is that strong willed, I think. It's funny, I used to know all these actors and I never hear from them. But my friends who are gay have *all* stuck around me, have all helped me get fed when I couldn't get out on my own. If I didn't have them I don't know where I'd be.

They did come through for me

Darnell Davis Most of the black men in Oakland and in San Francisco that I know of won't go get medical attention. They're where I was when I first started out, "Don't tell anybody." So when I found out I called my family up. They were the first people I told and they were *great*. It doesn't matter to them that I've chosen to live life as a homosexual and also as a gay black man dating a Caucasian man. Their attitude was, If this is important to him, then it's important to us. That's the way it should be across the board, but there are so many people out there that don't get that. And you get that a lot in the black community.

In terms of being black and gay in a black family, I find that the black woman is more compassionate in these areas than a lot of the black men. Basically, it's compassion and having a heart. I have brothers-in-law, I have nephews-in-law and they treated me with the greatest of respect. That's the true black man, not the black man that you see running around on the street, gang banging and carrying on like mad people. These are immature children; and those are people like any other race who are going to be critical and hard and have harsh words. Those are the ones you want to ignore. But my black people have treated me with respect and have come to my aid and have been there for me. I'll tell you, as a kid growing up I would have felt the opposite, 'cause that's how we were raised. "That's a faggot." And then here I was, and I loved it, you know, the respect that I got. They would never ever bad mouth me; they would never say anything bad about me. That's what the true black community's about: they care. When you get away from the nonsense and the stereotyping and the crap you see on TV.

AIDS in the heartland

Brad Sherbert I stayed at my mother's house out in the country near Hope. A few months after I got there, I moved into an AIDS residence which was one house kind of like the Shanti Houses used to be. I had to move there because Little Rock was the only place that had doctors that would see me. If I had a medical emergency, I didn't want to have to go 120 miles. Between where my mother lived and Little Rock there was not a doctor or a hospital that would touch me. Even my own doctor that I grew up with said, "Look, I'm not afraid of HIV but if word got out none of my other patients would come around." He was probably right 'cause the public was paranoid. Yeah, if I would've been seeing him having HIV, all his patients would've went somewheres else. I know they would've, no question about it.

But, yeah I moved into the AIDS residence in Little Rock. The house was six bedrooms with one person per bedroom. The house was never filled. There was no waiting list. We had one HIV support group on Monday nights and we had the AIDS Foundation, which did literally nothing. There was a clinic at the University of Arkansas Hospital for people with HIV every Thursday morning. It was a trip. Everybody had an appointment at like nine o'clock. They put us all in these little cubicles and then they'd gather our files and all the doctors would go back there and discuss everything. Then they'd come back and talk to us. We'd stand in the doorways of the cubicles while we were waiting for the doctors to come out of their meetings and we'd talk and stuff to each other 'cause PWAs were the only people there. Back then, in '88, I met people coming out of the smallest towns to that one clinic 'cause that was the only place in the state. So the clinic was pretty busy.

Arkansas families and HIV

As far as families, I was lucky. I had a very supportive mother. But as far as most people's families, it's like, just forget it. You're laid up in the hospital, you got AIDS, you're gay or you're a drug user, you made your bed and you've got to lie in it. I knew people with families right there in Little Rock and they wouldn't even come halfway across town to see their kids when they were dying 'cause they had AIDS.

And once you were in the hospital it wasn't much better. They were feeding people off of throw-away dishes. All the other patients ate off of regular dishes. PWAs ate off of throw-away dishes. You were on the fourth floor at the University of Arkansas Hospital. You had a red sign on your door, right there in the open: "CAUTION: BODY AND BLOOD: CAUTION," "WARNING: BODY FLUID AND BLOOD PRECAUTIONS."

Most people that I saw with AIDS, they'd lay up in the damn hospital. What's sad about it was my mother and two or three other mothers, that either had kids with AIDS or had kids that died and wanted to do something, they would go up to this fourth floor and chatted with the nurses and built a rapport with them. The nurses would go down the hallway and talk to everybody that had HIV and ask them if they'd like a visitor. And all of them said yeah, sure. These mothers would go and see these people and treat them just like they were their own kids, "if there's anything I can do for you, can I take you out for a walk," just anything that they could do for these people. They did it a couple of times a week. They formed a support group so they could talk about everything that they were seeing. And it was really quite neat. Well, the Arkansas AIDS Foundation started bashing them so they quit doing it because they didn't like all the shit they were catching for doing it. The Foundation was openly calling them things like, "Tragedy Seekers." That was hard on these mothers. I'd see them visiting with somebody they didn't even know real well who was in the final stages of the disease and they'd be crying and stuff. It was hard on them and they kept going. It meant a lot. They haven't had a visitor in a couple of days. They may be laying there depressed. But when they see you walk in the door they'll maybe sit up, put their robe on and get a little life into them. You know, it's good for them.

I did two interviews, one with the *Arkansas Democrat* and one with Channel Nine. They did like an hour-long documentary on me. They asked my mother, "How do you feel that your son came home with AIDS?" And she's like, "What do you mean? How do I feel?" She said, "You don't stop loving your kids just because they come home with AIDS. If you do, you never loved them in the first place."

Families, funerals, and a leather jacket

Peter Groubert *Having taken an old friend into his home to die, Peter Groubert was also faced with handling the funeral. He comments on the kind of family dynamics he encountered with a family which hadn't been there when Tim was dying but was more than ready to run the funeral.*
So, I was in charge. It was one hell of a thing with his parents, who were born-again Christians. They used to call him on the phone and make him crawl out of bed and get on his knees and pray. And he would sit there and shit on himself while he was kneeling and praying 'cause he had no control and crying, but he just couldn't say no to them. They came and visited once for about an hour – just wanted to look at him. They didn't care about him; they cared about his soul.

After he died, I called them to tell them that he had passed away and that I would send them copies of his death certificate. They said, "Well, what do we do now?" I said, "Well you don't do anything." "What about his body?" And I said, "Well that's been taken care of." "Well how are we going to have a ceremony?" "Well you go ahead and you have a ceremony." She says, "Are you having a ceremony down there?" "Yes, but it's for friends and you're not invited." And I said, "you didn't help him while he was alive. Why are you interested in him now that he is dead?" They wanted to know what he had left. I said, "Nothing, for you. Everything else has been given away." He hadn't talked to them in many, many years. His father disowned him when he found out that he was gay and refused to talk to him up until that day.

Brad Sherbert This jacket, I had been here for like a year and this belonged to one of the first friends that I had here. He got bronchial pneumonia and wasn't recovering. He was poor but his family were wealthy Mormons. And they gave him the full Mormon funeral. He said he wanted to be buried with this jacket but he said his family would never permit it. He told me to take the jacket before he died.

Families are funny when somebody dies. I had a friend just a few months ago who died and he and his lover had just bought a computer together for like $2000. His mother took the computer like the day the guy died, so his lover was like still in shock and couldn't stop her. They had each paid half. And what was most awful about this was that beside the computer was an ashtray the guy that died had made when he was like in kindergarten. The mother took the computer, didn't care nothing about the ashtray that her son had made. She knew it was there; she saw it and knew what it was; she wouldn't take that. That's how families get; they really do; they get greedy; they really do.

Robert Boulanget I hate that word, "family." I swear, I really do.

Black Panthers and evolving demographics

As the epidemic raged through the city, those who never thought they were at risk found themselves testing positive. Cynora Jones, an African-American woman, felt like life was finally all in place with her career and her family and then her husband got sick. Cynora didn't view herself as "the other." She let it all hang out during our hour-long interview, sometimes angry, sometimes crying. In a wavering tone modulating between excited and defeated, energetic and quiet, Cynora explained what the world looked like from the point of view of a black woman with HIV, as a person who has learned what it is like to be treated as a pariah.

Cynora Jones The story that needs to be told, I'm one of the stories. Let me tell you a little about myself. I'm forty-two years old. I'm a native San Franciscan. I'm one of the hidden population, the housewife. I came up during the '60s, during the '70s. What kind of a background? I went from being a Jehovah's Witness to a Black Panther to an executive of a 500 Corporation. I got married young. I was involved in a lot of things; I used drugs, was promiscuous, a lot of things.

About twelve years ago I decided I was really going to turn around a lot of things in my life. I got hired for a consulting firm. (*Laughs.*) The firm decided to merge with their other group in Glendale, California. I moved to Glendale in 19-something for my career. I was responsible for about $300,000 a week of the company's money. Life was beautiful.

In 1992, I was in a car accident in May and hurt myself pretty badly. And November of the same year my husband totaled out his car and he went to bed. About the same time I was getting up, he was going down. And things were happening to him that I just didn't understand. He was getting real moody, very mean, losing a lot of weight. We were arguing all the time and I didn't know why. I told him he needed to go to the doctor, "Something's wrong with you," and he would retort, "You need to go to the doctor." Anyway, it was really bad and getting worse. By the end of December I called his family.

I called the paramedics to the house three times, and because he could say who he was and what day it was, they wouldn't take him. It wasn't until after my in-laws came back on a mission to kidnap him, brought him back up to San Francisco and he passed out in the bathroom, that was the only way that he was admitted to the hospital. I talked to him on the phone first. He told me the doctor had told him he had food poisoning. So I flew up and one doctor told me, "We are admitting him as an AIDS patient," and I blew my mind. I was where everybody in life usually wants to be. I had the house, the cars, everything, and all of a sudden you're telling me my husband has AIDS?

Scared and recategorized, reclassified

This was in January of '93 and he was admitted. I was there every day. "You have AIDS," I tried to tell him. And at one point he says to me, "Why would you wish that upon me?" He was in total denial. He died in my arms February 22nd, 1993 and it wasn't because of the AIDS. I really do believe he died because everybody knew I was infected and the secret was out. I went back to Glendale in April.

I went back to the same clinic he, we had tested in. I really don't know what I was even testing for but I tested because he said I needed the test. I knew I had something, I didn't know what and the director could see I was so distraught. She said, "What's the matter?" I said, "Well Herbert's dead." She said, "What did he die from?" I said, "From AIDS." She said, "Well, you didn't know." I wanted to kill that woman, right there, I wanted to kill her. (*Tears begin.*) You can say I was diagnosed 1993 in March. In April I was diagnosed with full-blown AIDS. I've had a luxury of having HIV for a long long time.

How it affected me, um, I lost my mind, OK? (*Clears throat as tears pour*) and I told the people I work for. I bring this up because I work for a very prominent company. I had fifteen people up under me I was responsible for and a great deal of money every week. But when I told them that Herbert died from AIDS and I had it, I was demoted. I was like crazy then. I didn't even really understand what was going on. All my friends disappeared. My son, he had gotten a girl pregnant. Her parents made her abort the child because of my diagnosis. So within a few months I lost my life, my husband, a $106,000 a year job and my grandchild behind this epidemic. I was really pissed. For four months I went into a depression where I talked to my husband, drank and cried in my little room. I didn't want to be here. I wanted to die. I was scared to death. I used to wake up to see if I was still breathing, OK?!

I knew there was AIDS. I'd heard of AIDS, that it was a gay disease and definitely wasn't a black disease and it definitely wouldn't belong to me. I'm heterosexual and I'm having sex with one man, my husband, OK, my husband. Why would I protect myself from him? And I grew up with doctors. So eventually I guess somehow, like I said, I knew I had something . . . Here it is a little over two years and I'm just now starting to accept because, you know, I look back at it now and I was just nuts. I wanted to not look at it. I didn't want to be here.

The other and the institutional question

Brad Sherbert The main difference that I notice between here and living in Arkansas is I felt like a freak because everybody was paranoid, but out here it's no big deal. Psychologically, it's a lot better to have AIDS out here than in Arkansas. It was like being treated like a leper.

Even when I went to apply for my food stamps, they gave me a ten o'clock appointment. I showed up at ten o'clock. One o'clock in the afternoon, all the case workers had come back from lunch, I still hadn't seen anybody. They were takin' in people that had showed up after me with only a ten- or a fifteen-minute wait. If other people had been waiting there all day I would have just sat there 'cause I figured they've got more work than they can handle. But I'm sitting here waiting all day because some jerkwad case worker doesn't want to see somebody with AIDS. I went up to the window and its like, "I had a ten o'clock appointment." They gave me some kind of bullshit story what was taking so long. Finally I just hollered, "Look, God damn it, I've got AIDS. I'm sick. I don't have the fucking energy to sit here all day." When I said that, that office just cleared out. All the other clients went home and the case worker came out and said, "Well, I guess you're next." (*Laughs.*) Blatant discrimination: they knew that I was there to collect stamps because I had AIDS. And they didn't want to give them to me.

I've seen a lot of that. People still are afraid of people with AIDS. There's still a lot of attitude about, "Well, you deserve just what you got." There's a lot of that attitude. I'm sure it probably exists here just as it did in Arkansas. I'm hangin' around mostly the gay community here and they're pretty open to it but I bet it exists here too.

The impact of HIV on the family

Cynora Jones I'm telling you. I would liken the people that were in my surroundings to like if a person's ever lived in a house with roaches. If you walk in a room that has roaches, they scatter. That's what happened to people that said they loved me, OK, just like roaches. But I found another community now which keeps me going and that's women with HIV and AIDS and fuck what people think. In my insanity I started hooking up with a support group in Pasadena. It really just dawns on me now but I was the only person like myself at that support group because everybody else at that support group was white and gay. And it just now dawns on me a year and a half later, "Hey wait a minute, there was something wrong with that picture, OK." But if it hadn't been for the man I'm with now, he literally kidnapped me out of Glendale, literally, I'd have died there. Yeah, he packed me up literally.

Nobody could understand what the fuck happened, what the fuck was going on. We're a happy family and all of a sudden my daughter's got snatched out. She left, because, she, you know, "Dad's dying, Dad's dead, Mom's dying." In a matter of a few months the kids on my son's football team stopped talking to him, OK? A lot of people get affected by this. Why "the Other?" Fear and ignorance and I'm better than! That happens to those people and not myself. I was one of them. It couldn't happen to me. Fear and ignorance.

I'm pissed! How the hell are they going to tell me that; they would tell me that this man's got gonorrhea or syphilis, but if he's got a life threatening damn disease, they allowed him to kill me. If he'd had syphilis or gonorrhea, they could have contacted me but because of the fucking confidentiality law, they allowed my husband to kill me. If I was to go out and do the same damn thing knowing I have this disease and go out unprotected and have sex with someone and not tell them, I could go to jail. It's bad enough that he didn't have the courage to be able to tell me. I understand now and I have a lot of feelings about that. I still love him. I miss him very much. I hate him a lot many times. I also understand that he carried this disease, this secret by himself. He was suffering. He was suffering. He would rather die than have to deal with having AIDS. Do you see? He gave up. They told me when they admitted him, "He'll make it through this. This is his first bout. This is the first time he's ever got sick." He chose not to be here. He told me. I asked him, "What do you want to do, live or die?" He said, "Die." I said, "I'll stay here until you do." He didn't want anyone. He was a proud black man. He was a Muslim. How can he face the fact that he had AIDS? And on top of that he was systematically giving it to me. I remember like in retrospect him saying shit like, "In three years you're going to hate me." And I was thinking to myself, "I hate you right now. What the fuck are you talking about?"

The poverty of HIV and otherness

Hazel Betsey *Hazel recalled a failure to find the resources, personal and public, to take care of herself through a downward spiral into homelessness.* As far as AIDS went in Connecticut, I kept hearing that it affected homosexuals. I wanted to find some information around that because I was one, right? Then I thought, OK, lesbians were the safest category because we didn't screw men. I wasn't using so I wasn't going to get it through IV drugs. I didn't believe in blood transfusions so I was in a group that was of the elite, OK? (*Laughs.*) And I moved here to San Francisco and I started hearing the news that guys were dropping like flies here in this city, but I still felt that I was safe.

I got here and I worked for a youth hostel. Still, the AIDS thing just wasn't something that I thought about. When I started being sexually active I didn't practice safe sex at all. I would drink, get drunk, pick up somebody. I still thought that lesbians were safe until I had an affair with this woman for the weekend, a really young girl, like nineteen.

I was working at this gay bar at the time. About a month or so later, she came into the bar and she had tears in her eyes, right. I was like, "What's wrong?" She says, "I need to talk to you." "What's up?" She goes, "Well, I have AIDS. You need to go get tested." "What do you mean you have AIDS? You're a lesbian." She goes, "Well, I used to shoot up drugs."

I got in another relationship after that. This time I was homeless by choice because I was sick of, really, my addiction, and I wanted to do something different with my life. If I didn't have a job and I didn't have any money, I wouldn't buy any drugs. I was so naive. I didn't know anything about the world, that even being homeless and poor you can still have lots of sex and drugs. I didn't really look for it but I was around people that had it and they always gave it to me. This woman and I lived in a car down at China Basin. It was a big 1960 something station wagon. We started using a lot. I'm getting into where I was infected, this was in 19—? '88 and she went home for Thanksgiving.

Once she was gone I really started using a lot and I had an affair with this young guy; he was like eighteen or nineteen. I met him while I was out there hanging out. I just got hooked seeing him for that day so I said to him, "You're kind of attractive. We'll go have sex. (*Slaps back of hand against the other palm for emphasis.*) You have to use a condom." "I'm in the military," he responded. "We get tested all the time and you can't have HIV in the military. They'll throw you out." So I figure, "Hey, he's in the military." I was messed up. So he stayed with me that night.

About two weeks later, I got really sick, flu, diarrhoea. You know, I went to the doctors and the hospital. They never tested me for HIV. They looked in my lungs and this is what kind of pissed me off, the fact that they weren't testing women back then. If a man came in right away with those symptoms, they'd test him. This was '87, thousands had died. Anyway, they told me I had bronchitis and gave me antibiotics, big huge giant pink pills. So I took those and I still didn't think I was infected. You know, one thing this guy told me that he was bisexual, but the only thing I heard was that he was in the military and that he could not be infected. I didn't hear the other stuff.

I wanted to get away. This life was too crazy. At the same time my tonsils got huge. My voice was changing and it was hard for me to swallow. I went to this clinic there and they said, "Your tonsils may be infected. That could be cancerous and this and that." He wanted to run some tests including an HIV test. I looked at him, I was like, "You do?" He was like, "Yeah, let's just do it." I said, "OK," and it came back positive. "I'm positive?" and I didn't believe him.

A very specific group

Through the years, HIV has grown to increasingly affect America's greatest other, the urban poor (Fullilove, 1993; Timmons, 1996; Hilts, 1996A).

Ronnie Ashley Seventy percent of my clientele are women and children, African American women and Latino women, Native American women are dying faster than any population.

Per Eidspjeld I think it has something to do with education on the downfall. There's a lot of people who just don't know better; they never got any education. And that's a sort of politics and money and who gets what, who lives in what neighborhood. And it's protecting people, national security. If you are going to get real cynical about AIDS, I would go as far as to say it's an advantage to certain people in our society because those suffering from it are IV drug users, prostitutes, Latins, blacks and gay people. If these people are going to die off that's going to satisfy a bunch of other people who don't see themselves in these categories.

Richard Chavez This is a disease that is convenient to the society to stop population growth, to provide jobs for people. It's good for the economy.

Hazel Betsey I came out to this woman once that I was HIV-positive and she said, "I'm not surprised 'cause you used drugs and you're black. You're already a high risk category." I used to feel that because I was a black woman, I would get treated different. Like the doctors who said they weren't even surprised. They were like, "Yeah, well, you're in a high risk category." I thought, what the hell does that mean to be a woman and be a high risk category? I was doomed to destruction just because I am a black woman. I hate to say this but I know it's true. A lot of black women, I'm going to speak for women specifically out there who are infected, don't even know it. Some know it and don't care and they're having unsafe sex. I keep meeting women who are pregnant bringing infected babies into this world. I wish that a lot of black people wouldn't say that it's a white man's disease and that it's planted in the black communities, 'cause it's not. So I get angry at my own people when I hear them talk that way because it just keeps them back here. Instead of them saying, "I have it. I want to live and do what I can and help my children," they kind of ostracize themselves and say, "Them bastards infected me, fuck them. I'm going to live and I'm going to enjoy my life." What that means is "I'm not going to be safe. I'm not going to give a shit about anybody else." That's what's sad.

Incest

Many people with HIV, men and women, have incest backgrounds. During my two years of work at an AIDS housing program, clients consistently referred to childhoods of incest, followed by drug addiction preceding HIV infection. The cycle involves early invasion of the self, diminishing hope and belief in self, creating attitudes of low self-worth, and later in life high-risk behaviors leading to infection (McAdams, 1990; Bowlby, 1979; Elson, 1988; Alders, 1993; Zastrow and Ashman, 1995; Purnell, 1996). Drugs, as a means of escape, of course play a key role (Hilts, 1996A). Hazel relates her child abuse experience and its relation to her present life.

Hazel Betsey Total invasion: I think that a lot of people who are HIV-positive, those of us that have it who are young and if we were incest survivors, we started doing drugs. The incest eventually takes over and you can't deal with it. If you don't get in recovery around that when you are young, when you're older it is going to hit you. It hit me hardest when I got oldest. I dealt with it when I was young and I survived it, whatever way I knew. But when I got older it really hit me and I started doing more drugs around it. And if I thought about it and I felt worthless, I felt like I never was going to fit in anywhere, like I could never marry a man. I could never feel safe in sex with a man, ever. I tried and I didn't. I had sex with women much more but then I ended up getting infected by a man because I was using.

I was staying in a bus. I was high and I didn't want to stay alone that night. If I was in my right head I would have insisted on getting condoms. A lot of gay men that are infected were heavy drug users and just didn't practice safe sex. And a lot of women that are infected in my recovery groups didn't practice safe sex, were incest survivors and used drugs heavily 'cause they were affected. It's very few people that I run into that got HIV that never used drugs, that lived these little normal lives and were never incest, were never molested. Few that got it that way through the blood transfusions. The majority of us definitely had something taken away and just went towards that life, was led in that direction, didn't know how to get in recovery around any of our issues.

A lot of us that are in recovery now say, "I'm not in recovery because of my HIV status; I'm in HIV because my life was fucked up and I got sick of it. I got sick of feeling the pain." When I started feeling the pain of my child abuse, I always ran away. I didn't know how to deal with it so when it got powerful, when it really ate at me and I started feeling like I didn't fit in where I was at, I moved because that was the easiest way to deal, go somewhere else and start life all over again. Maybe it will be different. Maybe you will meet some different people. Maybe you will feel different about yourself. And I did for a little while. I liked the newness, but eventually it came down to those same feelings. When I came to San Francisco, I knew something had to change and the first thing I had to change was my addiction.

Stresses on family relationships

Paul Greenbaum   In terms of my romantic relationships, there's no question that HIV affects your or other people's desire for being involved with each other. Someone may not want to get involved with you because you're HIV-positive and they, they themselves may be positive. More likely in that situation they'd be negative but they may not want to deal with loss. Who's going to die first? I have a boyfriend. He's HIV-positive; he's an AIDS widow. His lover died about two to three years ago which is recent, very recent, and he's twenty-nine. Intimacy can be a problem, nevertheless. He's been through one loss; I've not been through a lover but more roommates, friends, and acquaintances than I care to think about have died. It's hard to become friends with someone knowing that you may outlive them. But I've never let that deter me. I've decided just to hang in there and endure the loss.

My last roommate was also positive. Towards the end, before he moved back home, most of the time that we spent together was going to and from the doctors. But I'm glad that I had the chance to help him. I'm not into Judgment Day or any of that, but when the time comes I would put that as a little feather in my cap, that I helped this guy. It's changed my relationships. I'd rather have five good friends than ten casual friends. I'm much more focused on melding good relationships and less concerned about the things that don't matter that much. It's certainly taken me away from some of the superficiality.

Hugo Manzo I didn't tell you about what happened over the holidays did I? Well, I was in Houston and I was staying in with an old friend. I get a lot more attention in Texas than I do here. I had five guys wanting to buy me drinks one of those nights at the bars. The whole thing was very good for my ego. I can barely get a date when I am here. It is very difficult. Here, all anybody looks at is the face and the body. I have an ugly face and an ugly body so nobody looks at me. San Francisco is hard on people. Not many people do find anyone. People are selfish or scared. In San Francisco, people only look to people to help them. They only befriend people who can help them get what they want. But I do understand the fear. I am scared to have sex. I do not want to get reinfected or to infect anyone else.

I just don't think about men. Instead I just give Manuela (*Hugo gestures at his right hand with a smile*) a call every day. And we gay men always have the cruising park. It's better than the sex clubs and the locker rooms. It's free, why not? Plus it's cleaner. Those other places, the smell, I cannot stand it. It's like somebody died.

Art It's been very difficult, and sometimes it's OK and sometimes it's overwhelming. If I am in a place that's at all prone to depression, there it goes and it can really pull me away. I went through a series, a few years ago at the beginning of this thing, of people who would not involve themselves in a relationship with me because they were afraid I was going to die. Now they're all dead. I had a lot of sadness and rage about that for a while. It hasn't happened for over six years, but when it did, it was like one after another and "Oh no, this just scares me too much, blah,

blah, blah . . ." And then they got sick and died. This was a few people, not just a handful, but a group.

Sometimes one doesn't fall in love again. I just ended a relationship that was not at all healthy; but before that there hadn't been anything in a while and I don't know as there will be anything in the near future or ever. You know it can be a very treacherous kind of thing, how people deal with health issues and their motivation. I run across a lot of caretakers, drama queens. It's not an easy thing. I'm not saying it should be. I don't know how much of that is illness related and how much of that is just dealing with what I have had to deal with, my health and facing things that I really require other people to face as well or there's no relationship. I can't have a good time relationship with someone who can't meet me wherever it is that I am.

"I'm gonna take care of you. You need me don't you?" (*Sounding very prissy.*) That kind of thing. That was part of my last relationship. I was this lover, AIDS patient, and we talked about it a number of times and I said, "You know, this isn't going to work and I'm not going to play this drama." I said, "No, no, no, no, no, no." And he never got it. He needed that drama very badly. He was sending out resumés for jobs and on the top was an objective copping out on his own future and not fulfilling his own potential. "I am not looking for something to fulfil my career goals but to pay a few bills so I can spend time with my lover." He put this on his resumé. What the hell would you do with that? What kind of story can you tell an employer from such dramatics? I really didn't end up caring to be part of the drama on that.

It's common with relationships, among caregivers. At the hospice it wasn't the people who were dying who were a stress, it was the people who were coming to help them. They were getting their identity and their life from somebody else's suffering. A lot of people never look at why they are doing this. I am not copping to the things they are getting from senses of being needed and being loved and being wanted, self-satisfaction and ego things, drama and avoidance of their own personal issues, of their own pain and growth. "Oh no, he's dying. Look what I can do for him. You need me don't you?" "No, I don't. Maybe I need you to be you. That would be great." You can use everything for your own personal good, but don't call it something else. Don't go into martyrhood or into self-pitying about it. You've got some stuff going too. Honestly, you should have some sort of an idea of what it is.

TWELVE

Lives within a Model

ACT UP was by no means the only form of activism to take on the epidemic during the 1980s. Many organizations such as Cleve's KS (later dubbed AIDS) Foundation, Project Inform, Project Open Hand and Shanti Project were created by people gathering together in response to the epidemic. This network of grass roots groups has been dubbed "the San Francisco Model," (Fernandez, 1991). In 1990, resources allocated for the Ryan White Care Act were provided to create service systems across the country based on this model (Hilts, 1990). The following is a look at the issues, ins, outs and world views of PWAs both involved as clients receiving services from and volunteering with these organizations.

Ronnie Ashley In '85, I just told Kurt, "I want to sell the businesses and I want to get out of Texas 'cause I want to know what the hell is going to happen to me." The only news that was coming out was coming out of San Francisco. You were hearing about people consistently hitting the streets and protesting. You heard these horror stories on TV as far as, "Oh, fags in San Francisco and what they were making." I wanted to come to San Francisco because I wanted to find out more about HIV, but yet, at the same time, deep in our guts we both knew also that politically San Francisco was the place to be.

Intellectual activism – the world of Project Inform

Paul Greenbaum The AIDS diagnosis was a real kick in the pants, that led me into the treatment movement. Then I realized more than ever that I was part of a despised minority. I got started on the AIDS Foundation Hotline which was OK. I ended talking to what they call "the worried well." It wasn't the audience I wanted to reach. But I did make some contacts and learned more about Project Inform and ACT UP and those types of organizations and gradually gravitated over the next year. There was a man who was a long-term AIDS survivor, which in 1987 was no mean feat, and he made a series of four or five like seven-hour workshops on how to successfully have AIDS and live with it. He wrote the first book that I read on the subject, *Living with AIDS*. It was definitive at the time. He was a link to the treatment underground.

No matter how much of an activist I am, I have always been an intellectual activist. My activism has been with stuff such as Project Inform, which actually is being quite a bit of an activist compared to organizations which are mostly into providing services such as Open Hand. I don't criticize them. That's a form of activism, but it's not as focused politically like being with Project Inform or ACT UP. There you're not just helping people, you're saying, "The price of this drug is too high or the access is too restricted." I may not have participated in negotiating with pharmaceutical companies or picketing, but working on the hotline has been more my way and it's also forced me to keep up on this volume of reading. I don't know if you noticed all these notebooks on my desk. There are all these different newsletters. That brown box over there is full of stuff that I had to create manila folders for, because everything I have had, a file for AZT, DDI. That's been my involvement.

Jay Segal The new reality is ongoing from Project Inform who I consider part of the cutting edge. We know the next set of questions to be asked. We know where things are going. And there are some really cool "Gods" as I call them there in terms of writing and research. There was Jesse Dobson. He made people who wouldn't normally talk about this sit down for two days and say, "Thank you, we want to do more of this. We really accomplished a lot." It started some trials and the beginning of genetic engineering; it got some people together. They aren't doctors. They aren't people who have money behind them. These are scientists talking together and they want to share. These are people from Africa, people from Australia, people from Europe, the top in the world, Jonas Salk, Gallo, Montagnier, the people with the names and the history. Then we had the ACT UP kings and queens from the world. We had the activists, although Project Inform is actually considered an activist organization. We had everybody there in a think tank.

They were given two questions, one per day. In your hands, you have a cure for AIDS. What do you do with it? I want to hear a plan, every single detail from step one to the finish. And how are you going to do it? How are you going to jump over Congress? How are you going to jump over society and its hatred of this disease? How are you going to jump over that fact that people aren't going to want to get a shot of AIDS vaccine because they are going to be afraid they catch AIDS? They brainstormed and came up with some really neat answers. There have been two immune restorations think tanks; the third one is in planning. Jesse Dobson who organized this had no T-cells, no immune system left.

Tales from the Emergency Fund

Dan Vojir I've been with the AIDS Emergency Fund for almost four and a half years. When I wanted to do some volunteer work, one of my criteria was I work for an organization that's not so big that the proceeds just go to organizational work. Then only 30 or 40 percent go back to the clients. AIDS Emergency Fund was all volunteers, and still is to a degree because we have like three paid staff people. But almost 90 percent of the dollars still go to the services, still go directly to the clients. We pay their bills. We pay their hospital, whatever . . .

I went to the office and they needed it at the time and I started doing client intake. You could go pick up penny jars around the city or sponsor a beer bust, but client intake was a hell of a lot different. You see those people. I was trying to do it two afternoons a week and I started burning out. When I went in I was hoping that maybe they would have something for me to do on the computers in the back. I would see this look on the manager's face like, "Guess what? You're the only one that came in this afternoon." I had this weird karma. You could ask the former manager, Chris. He said, "We could have the quietest afternoon, no one comes in or very few, it's nice. Dan comes in and all hell breaks loose; the weirdest cases in the world seem to gravitate to you." He says, "I don't know why, but with you it is just absolutely awful." It's true, I would get all these bizarre cases.

I got a case once where I answered the phone and hear: "You gotta help me. The guys outside my house are trying to disconnect my PG&E." And it was cold. "I've just come back from the hospice." I said, "Well, did you apply to have us pay it because maybe they just haven't gotten a check yet?" "No." Oh God. He was a client, thankfully, but he hadn't applied to have the bill paid. There was the money in the account to pay the bill. He just hadn't told us to pay it. I said, "Wait just a minute, OK?" I asked the client I was with to wait a few minutes. A couple of frantic calls, one fax and it was over within twenty minutes. The dispatcher was called and told to get off of his front lawn. It was getting paid. What a close call though, because once he did get disconnected, he wouldn't have had enough money to get it reconnected.

I have been at the desk when we had both a mother and a son diagnosed. I had one fourteen-month-old kid who made a real impression on me. He was just beginning to walk and he had full-blown AIDS; his mother had full-blown AIDS also. That's hard, that's difficult. I saw one kid who was two years old and already had two bouts of pancreatitis. The kid did not smile, even when he was feeling good. This is true. His mother was positive and knew she had AIDS when she conceived but had the child anyway. She just wanted the kid. She was very selfish and, of course, she died right after he was born. Just a total selfish act. This little kid, for the first two years of his life had to suffer for it 'cause the mother wanted the child. I don't know if he's still living.

Every week, it's my reality check. I'm on the board of directors now but I still try to do client intake whenever I can. Everybody should have something where they know somebody else is a hell of a lot worse off than they are. We used to have one guy where we had paid his rent. Every month he came in with a box of donuts on the anniversary of the rent check because he said, "If it weren't for you guys I wouldn't have my apartment." It's all he could afford but every month he would come in with a box of donuts.

Hugo Manzo Volunteering was a beautiful experience. If I had to do this again, I would do the same thing 'cause I learned so much about the disease. It actually was helping me to understand myself more and to accept myself more. It gave me a lot of, not power, but empowerment to keep on living. It has been my medicine for actually being alive after being HIV-positive for such a long time without taking medications.

When I was volunteering I lost 150 clients. They were friends; I don't see them as clients. After losing so many friends, I had to step back because I was harming myself. I was not getting the support to continue. I would just go by their houses and give them emotional support or if they were too sick to do anything, I would help them clean their house, cook for them or just accompany them to the hospital for appointments. Most of the time I was helpful as a translator.

One client, Jose Louis, La Coca-Cola, was a very special relationship. I knew him for two years. He was a stubborn person. He used to call me a frustrated philosopher and sometimes he kicked me out of his house because I would not agree with him on things. I would suggest to him not to take medicines that would harm his body or not agree with things that he will say. I will argue especially when it comes to spirituality. He was a recovered alcoholic for ten years and he was very rooted into his system of being free from drugs from AA. I think that AA gave him life again, but at the same time it made him a very selfish person. For me it was an issue of showing him the thing was not about being self-centered. It was about giving. Fifteen days before he died I threw a birthday party for him and that was my victory. He finally gave in and told me that I was . . . (*Hugo's eyes well up; he rubs them and pauses.*) I can't believe this is going to make me cry after two years. He told me I was one of the best persons he had ever met his whole life, a person that really gives himself to his friends and he thanked me for never stopping going to his house after he kicked me out of his house for so many times.

You know, it's sad to lose so many friends. I try not to remember any more. It's too sad for me. This epidemic has gone too far. There's a lot of pain and there has already been a lot of suffering. I try not to think about it. And when I do I try to laugh about it, big jokes. Being sarcastic sometimes helps you in dealing with your own disease.

Strength in numbers

Philip Blazer   Just before my first illness, I wanted to make sure that I had everything taken care of so that when I'm sick and really need something the bank would come over with food, Project Open Hand. I had such a great group of friends as far as bringing meals. They all had a day and all knew to call to check on me. I said, "Don't go to any trouble, save your leftovers." I love to eat, I'd eat anything. I really didn't have to utilize a lot of the community services I was signed up for. They were there, "We just wanted to make sure." That was great.

It's safety in numbers. Whenever I have gone to a support group, to a seminar, or to a presentation I always feel better about the sense of me not being the only one than I have from the information from the meeting. Say they were talking about wasting syndrome. The fact that I went and talked, can see others there, and talk to them and feel I'm not alone. I get such a good reinforced positive feeling. I've felt that from the start, so I try to involve as many other people as I can.

Hazel Betsey   *She compares and contrasts the resources she used in New Jersey to those in San Francisco.* It started getting really hard being in the closet, really emotionally draining. Every time I would go to the clinic, I would have a different doctor. It was all these interns and half the time they didn't even read my file. They didn't even know I was infected. So I got really turned off by the clinic. They wanted to put me on AZT, they thought I was foolish that I didn't want to go on it. I told them about my side effects, I don't want to do it. I was always trying to find a good doctor that I could feel safe with. I could never find it. So I knew I needed to get out of New Jersey. Nobody ever talked about AIDS and if they did, it was always negative. It was a small town. It was just not the place to be if you're infected. So I left.

I had a feeling that San Francisco was the place to be because I felt like they were probably doing a lot of research here and they must be really up on this disease by now. So I came here on New Year's Eve, '94. In January, I went to Lyon Martin's clinic, got a low T-cell count. I started reading everything I could get my hands on. I have this particular book that I got attached to, Kaiser's (1993) *Immune Power*, and started following all the advice about writing letters to your disease, just communicating with it. I started therapy, got myself involved with this vitamin program, started acupuncture and Chinese herbs. I go to support groups, that's the most important thing.

At first I didn't look for women's groups. I didn't think they existed for some reason. You know, I thought I was the only one. When I went to recovery groups for people with HIV, it was men. I thought this was safe for me because I don't have any issues with gay men. We all have something in common, disease. But the stuff they talked about was not relating to me. They were mostly gay men, 90 percent of them were gay men. And this is not for me here either. So Lyon Martin started this group for women and I started going to that. Then I started finding women's recovery groups and I was just so excited. I do that twice a week. I started to hear how many women in recovery were also HIV.

In the end

Philip Blazer It's a crisis among us. I don't want to say my people, like the gay people have the exclusive right on this disease, but my neighbors, my co-workers, my family here. It's affected us. You have to; I just cannot see not getting involved. The second most important single form of support other than my family has been the community out here.

THIRTEEN

WORLD

In 1990 Rebecca Denison went with a friend to get HIV tests back. She turned out to be the one who tested positive. When her husband tested negative, she called a boyfriend of six years prior. He was already dead. She searched for support mechanisms. Groups for men abounded; only one support group served women with AIDS. She did not qualify because she had HIV, not AIDS. In response, Denison, with help from ACT UP, set up WORLD: Women Organized to Respond to Life-threatening Diseases. She started a newsletter which has found huge popularity. WORLD now puts on retreats, offers classes on women and HIV, and most importantly provides a network for those with a disease which has become the third largest killer of women, aged twenty-five to forty, in the country (Hilts, 1996A). WORLD is reflective of women's response to the radically shifting demographics of HIV disease (Denison, 1995). The following are stories of women involved in and around WORLD.

Although the CDC statistics are clear – AIDS is the leading cause of death for all Americans aged twenty-five to forty-four (Weir, 1995) – the world still views HIV as a gay male disease. This is partly because the speed with which the face of AIDS evolves eludes easy categorization. Although the first phase of HIV was among gay white men, the epidemic is having a disproportionate effect on the black and Latin populations (Fullilove, 1993; McDaniel and London, 1995) and women (Shaw, 1993). Women suffered large increases in 1994, the most recent year for which such statistics are available. There was a 30 percent increase in AIDS deaths among white women, a 28 percent increase among black women. AIDS caused one in five deaths of black women aged twenty-five to forty-four (Hilts, 1996A).

The problems women endure, with AIDS, as with the case of many situations for women in our culture, remain buried in the closet where the dominant culture does not see them. I had a great deal of trouble finding HIV-positive women willing to speak publicly. Part of this problem stems from the stigma still surrounding the disease. One HIV-positive woman explained that she felt women are still labeled as stupid for becoming positive. It looks like they did not care about using condoms or shared needles. Another woman explained that when she disclosed her HIV status to her boyfriend, he called her a pariah.

The following women told me their stories and how they became involved with WORLD. They shared insights into how HIV disease highlights previously existing elements of sexism, racism, and classism within our society. Interviewees concluded with a discussion about the visibility of women with HIV and how best to continue their lives.

Yvonne Knuckles met me at WORLD in Oakland. WORLD banners hang everywhere. Rebecca Denison greeted us. Yvonne, a dark-skinned African-American woman, sat down, her brown braided hair pulled back, wearing earrings, a blue jacket, black jeans and a button-up black shirt. In a calm cadence, using eye contact, this fifty-seven-year-old woman shared tales of a year in prison with HIV, transformations, and of the ways people benefit by coming out and telling their stories.

Yvonne Knuckles I'm from West Oakland. I was born in Arkansas but I came here when I was three and I'm known as Bunny. I had kids when I was seventeen. And I'm HIV-positive. I've known since '89. I was an IV drug user, used for like thirty-two years and I've been to prison three or four times.

This one particular time I got out of jail in '84 or something, my sister came and told me I needed to take an AIDS test. I knew nothing about AIDS. I'd heard of AIDS but, "Oh well I don't need to know about that. She's a liar." I didn't want to believe that I could catch it 'cause I had been using it all these years. I went on and I went back to prison and I came back again in '89. I was on parole. I had messed around and got hooked on heroin again. My parole officer called me so I had to tell her. This way she put me on methadone; that was when I tested.

I kept coming back and I found out nearly a month later. I said, "I've been walking around with this card." He took it and asked me if I would mind going in another room. The nurse was sitting there. She would talk to me. I hadn't thought 'cause I'm in a hurry, I want my methadone so I can get out of there. When I went in there to sit down, this lady looked up to me, "Oh, you know, you tested positive. You have AIDS." And when she said I had AIDS, I said, "Bitch, you're lying." I said, "You got to be crazy." You know, I just went off.

I break out of her office, right. Now I'm just thinking, I'm fixing to die and I knew I was going to die because this was all I knew. AIDS to me meant that you are going to die. It means you didn't have but a few days to live. I go upstairs and break into my counselor's office. I'm stammering, screaming. People are wondering what's wrong with me. I can't really say it, right? She has a client right in there with her so she left. I told her I needed to talk, now, and I told her, "I got AIDS." She says, "What?" I was lost. This lady told me, "Well what I could do is up your methadone. Give you a larger dose." I could get that anyway. At that moment I needed someone to tell me I wasn't going to die.

This guy that I arrive with, he's my good friend. He would give me a ride every morning to get my methadone. When I come out I'm crying and I started walking away from the car. He says, "What's wrong with you?" I'm screaming, crying and I can't tell him. If I go ahead and if I tell him that I have AIDS does he not want me to get back into his car? I'm going to have to catch the bus. I'm just through with life. It's over for me. I said, "Man, I got AIDS. I'm fixin' to die." He said, "What are you going to do?" He grabbed me and hugged me. I was an IV drug user and had shared many needles of many people. I called my sister and she said, "You're positive, right?" "Yeah."

It was like a fear. How many people did I did I give it to? I had a little baby boy born, a crack baby. That's why I didn't want to just come out and say, "I'm HIV. I have AIDS." All this stuff going through my mind, I didn't stop using; I started using more. I smoked crack; I drank all day. As much as I could get I would use. And I started pulling away, doing everything by myself. I was dealing drugs. I told them things like, "Well, they say I have AIDS so you guys can't use my outfit anymore." I didn't know about bleach or none of that stuff. I'm being truthful. I knew some people that came by and said, "John got AIDS. This other person got AIDS." Oh well it's not going to bother me.

Nancy Lemoins *Nancy, another woman who accesses WORLD, told me about the dynamics of her life and history from 1950s St. Louis to the 1970s West Coast counter-culture through drugs and the '90s.* I'm from one of those tricky backgrounds that looks really good on paper but it's kind of fucked up in reality. I actually started being insane when I was about thirteen. When I was in seventh grade I did LSD every day for six months. (*Laughs.*) My brother and I used to set our alarms for like six o'clock in the morning and wake up, take a hit of acid and go back to sleep and wake up just tripping. My parents were kind of freaked out. They proceeded to go nuts and I ran away a lot.

I fell in love with this woman when we were like sixteen. I think about that, we were totally out; we used to sit in the lounge at school and like hold hands and stuff. I don't know what we were thinking. I guess it just never occurred to us that we shouldn't. We graduated from high school a year early in '73 and moved together to the University of Washington. And I discovered there were all these other women. It was just a really amazing thing for me. I just felt like it was my job to sleep with every one, (*laughs*) men, women, you know, boys, girls, cats.

I was like such a lesbian separatist at the time, not a separatist but I really didn't hang out with men much. The women's community was really intense there at that time. In Olympia, there's that riot girl thing. It was really like that except that we were sort of like hippies. I just totally played sports, had sex, went to school, except I would do drugs occasionally. There were some women's bars I used to go to a lot. Really kind of a café scene a long time ago. I spent like hours; I used to sit in cafés, kind of meet people. It was an interesting time. We were all total addicts. It's like a time when everybody did drugs because it was accepted. Nobody said, "Don't do that." That's how I ultimately ended up getting positive. Well actually I was sleeping with men too. I really liked my life then but I wouldn't want to live it again.

So we moved back to Europe. It was kind of an excuse but it was also really my major disillusionment. I couldn't believe it was happening. I shouldn't have gone. We spent a lot of time in England and in Paris but then I got to Amsterdam and I got really stuck. I just started to shoot massive amounts of heroin. I don't even remember that entire six months. My friends got me out. So we went to England and I kicked heroin. I really felt like I saw this darkness in myself that I really (*blows air out of her mouth*), really just couldn't handle.

So I swore off drugs and I moved back to Seattle where I had this amazing attraction to this very fucked up horrible person. It was a very fucked up time in my life. I just was really out of control. I was chef and was embezzling a lot of money from the restaurant and we kind of turned to a life of crime. We moved back down here 'cause we were running away from the law and she got arrested and put in jail.

Crime and punishment, prison and HIV

Yvonne Knuckles I got out in '89 and I went right back because of selling drugs. I wasn't afraid of going to prison but I was more afraid this time I went 'cause they had told me I had the virus. I'm not saying that I got it. I hadn't tried to find out nothing 'cause I was fixing to die. They sent me over to CIW, California Institutional Women. Over there you're in a special unit, Walker A, just for women.

It held forty women. In the yard, it was like thousands. This was prison. You know, they got like two or three thousand women in prison. Forty of us were in one unit. They had rooms, like twenty rooms, two to a room. All the women back there have the virus. Some are very, very sick. I've seen people die back there. I was scared to death. When I got in there I seen some women that I knew. I didn't know they had the virus until I got there. I was able to talk to 'em some but I was just in the wrong place. You know I don't have this when I look at me. When I went to jail I was all small and black and sunken and things on me where I had been picking. I wouldn't talk about it.

We couldn't go in the yard with the main population. For a long time, maybe a whole year, they kept us locked there. When people would come in they would want us to go in our rooms and stuff. It was like people would have put a monkey in a cage and people come by and there's doors all around you. And you can't go in or out no place, but anybody coming by can peek in at you. When they would touch the door, they would take it and use something, not their naked hands.

You know, women fight in prison. If there was blood, we would have to take care of the person. The seals wouldn't touch 'em unless they was full bodied down. We didn't have an AIDS specialist, just a regular doctor in the clinic that served everyone on the yard.

Before the AIDS specialist came, people were walking like zombies back there. This first doctor, he didn't know a lot about it, not as much as me, seemed like. They put me on AZT although my T-cells were really high and I didn't need it. He gave everybody AZT. When you went in, you got AZT when you go to jail. And it just did a job on me. I turned black, really black. All my finger nails turned jet black. There were so many things happening in prison, it makes you feel like . . .

In jail it's cold to have the virus. People do you bad. There are a lot of timid people in jail that's not out like me. I've been going to jail so long that you don't say certain things to me because I'm known in jail. When I went back to prison, before I got to Walker A, I went through Sonora County Jail first, right. I had a hard time. People were wondering, the women were like, "Why are you taking that pill? Why are you always going out? Why the doctor always want to see you?"

Any time you lived in Walker A, everyone else knows you have HIV/AIDS. If you could find someone, they would let you move out there. But most of the women that I seen that went out, they all came back. A friend would say, "Oh, you got Bunny living in the room and she got AIDS man and you ain't afraid. You know, you're going to get it too."

They didn't know a lot about it on the yard. When you got AIDS, they say, "Here come those women, they got the shit." We started coming through the yard, "Here we come. We got the shit! y'all!" Everyone on the yard wasn't like that, but you have a lot of people that, like today, still have the fear.

Transformations

A doctor came in with the ACLU. He was a great doctor there for women. They came and they talked for us and we were able to go in the yard. We were able to go after functions. We started having education literature. I started going to Bible study. These two ladies would come a long way, every Wednesday. I kept telling them about my problems and how I was feeling and I kept thinking that God had given me this disease and stuff. I learned right there and then that he didn't and she told me that I needed to pray. I got an awakening that I could live. I think the Lord maybe spoke to me in prison because one day I was in my room and it was like, "Well don't turn the TV on Bunny, just talk to me. You gotta come up out of this room. You gotta go on with your life and you can live. You got a long life ahead and there are things out there that you can do to help people." For about thirty minutes I was sitting in my room just listening.

There was a girl who had been there before me. She had had AIDS a long time so I started talking to her, you know. She stood out a lot 'cause she knew a lot about it 'cause she read everything. Yeah, there was more than one that was really outstanding like that. It was a few back there that knew all kinds of stuff about the virus.

The ladies on the yard weren't afraid of us. People wanted to know too. There were a bunch of us there that were going out talking about it. A lot of ladies back there that knew a lot of stuff. I just didn't find out 'cause I was one of those people in rebellion. Once I found out or accepted it, then I started learning. There was a girl that knew about WORLD. She got the address from somewhere and we started getting the newsletter and all this information. We would pass it out around.

After prison

Then since I came out from prison I started going around to support groups, to the clinic and I didn't use. God changed me. I prayed and I was told like by some ladies that did Bible studies that you just got to give it to God and you can live with it. When I left prison everyone said

I would be back because I've been in and out of prison and in and out of Santa Rita all my life. Nothing had changed me. Programs, methadone, none of that had stopped me. When I accepted Christ, I just asked him, "Lord I need deliverance. I want to live." I didn't want to be on the street, come out and get back. I'm in good health. I have normal T-cells. It's nothing wrong with me but old age.

My family loves me. I'm the oldest person in my family in Oakland.

Distinctiveness of HIV for women

Cynora Jones We are very different. We have different diseases. We have different things happen. I get recurring breast infections. This is something totally new to my nurse practitioner because they have just now started doing studies on how it really infects women. And here I am, someone who is having consistent breast infections. This is my opportunistic disease, even though there is nothing written that says this is an opportunistic disease. But because I still have breast milk, my body is reacting this way. This is new. My nurse practitioner says "I have no one like you." When it first started happening I had a doctor ask me, "Oh, is that an abscess?" He assumed that I was shooting dope into my breast, OK! Doctors, same old story. Same old shit.

Hazel Betsey As far as medical goes, one thing that bothered me, but that's changing, is that a lot of the time in the clinical trials at the beginning were for men. So they were doing all these tests on men. So they had all this data about diseases that men would get and information and preventative measures. Whereas for women it didn't seem like they had that because they weren't doing any trials on us. There was no research. Like with SSI, the complications for SSI were male related diseases. If you look at it, "Have you ever had this, this, this?" "No, No, No." "Well then you're fine." So now that's changing.

Marija Mrdjenovic As far as the point of view of a woman, the best way to organize it would be, let's talk about T-cells. Men and women have differing T-cells. They do differ, by significant numbers. In 1987, I had 294 T-cells. By, I think, 1989 or so, I was down to below 200. So technically then, I had AIDS. But that definition did not exist yet. I had two T-cells last year, and now I have seven. Obviously something more is involved than just T-cells. A lot of people with sarcoma have T-cells of up to 700 yet they've got the lesions all over their face. With women, because you can have a lower T-cell count and that there is something else at play, the medical community doesn't recognize that.

There was no special consideration given to women's problems like cervical cancer, like cervical problems. They could happen outside of HIV, but nobody began to suspect that they could be triggered by it. For years, nobody suggested that. That's why women could get really *bad* cases of AIDS and then finally get treated. Even though the doctors knew they were HIV, they were seeing these gynecological problems, they still were not treating these women. They were always waiting for what I call crisis management.

The other problem is that women are expected to get the same illnesses as men. Sarcoma, for example, which was such an obvious condition and which had been diagnosed and thoroughly talked about, rarely happened in women. A lot of the illnesses like wasting syndrome were happening in the men, but they, as has just now been discovered, do not happen all that much in women.

Women's support mechanisms

Nancy Lemoins You know, retrospectively I realize that people had AIDS in the '80s. The first consciousness I had of AIDS was when I got HIV. I kind of knew I was positive because I kept getting these skin infections. I tested in '86 and they referred me to this place called ASAP, AIDS Substance Abuse Project. I went there and they were real idiots. None of the places I went at that time were very together. It wasn't till about '90 or '91 that I started accessing any services.

Lesbians were like, it was just implicit in a lesbian being HIV that you've been doing sort of taboo things. You know, either having sex with men or using IV drugs which really really was more prevalent in the lesbian community than anybody wants to admit. Really, it was very disillusioning. For me, I just was like, "Uhh, fucking assholes." I had a lot of my friends absolutely turn their backs on me. And I'm sure that really increased my paranoia so to speak. I never really was in the closet about this. I'm a lot more outspoken about it now.

I was like this militant lesbian for a while in college. I really identified with the lesbian community. Now I really kinda don't identify with them. More because I know a few lesbians who have HIV, but gay men and straight women have been a lot more accessible to me. I don't really have that many lesbian friends any more.

Hazel Betsey Socially, it's not a lot. I happen to be around a lot of straight women with the disease 'cause I can't find a lot of lesbians. Sometimes I feel like I'm the only one. Or maybe, I know of two others. I know seventy-five straight women. So sometimes I feel like I need a place to go where there's lesbians with HIV, a group or something. I feel like I'm totally invisible in the lesbian community. Anyway, I was asked to speak for lesbians with HIV at the dyke march before Gay Pride and to speak for lesbians with HIV which I did. It was very difficult for me but I did it.

I just talked about how lesbians with HIV have been treated invisible in this society around AIDS. After I got off stage this woman, it was like a three-minute speech, this woman jumped in my face and says, "Where do you get your data, your information!" I had mentioned that HIV can be transmitted from female to female contact. She says, angry, "Where do you get your information about female to female transmissions. This is not a fact. Where is that written?" And it just shocked me because I was talking about women practicing safe sex with each other. Don't take it for granted that you're a lesbian and you're safe. You're not any more. I know women that were infected by other women. I tell you, I know for a fact that a majority of lesbians are not practicing safe sex. I don't know, body fluids are body fluids to me.

Beyond "Why me?"

Marija Mrdjenovic A lot of women are still stuck in the "Why me?" stage. The women I've talked to are either depressed about their health and not ready to do anything about it or are so involved in the political side that they don't see that the answers are in immunology. They just see them as if we just push this senator or the FDA enough, they'll come up with an answer. But nobody, nobody, has really sat down and said, "We need gene therapy. We need to make these bodies healthy again." I feel very much alone around a lot of the women with HIV. I think a lot of them are so damned sure they're going to die. Most of the letters sent to WORLD are all about "poor pitiful me." I know that needs to be said by women that do feel alone, and I know that that's an important sort of step. But after seven years of reading nothing but "poor pitiful me," I just really want to say, "Well, wake up honey, smell the coffee; let's get together and let's force our opinion on these doctors." It's just not happening. The AIDS Coalition established by gay men is so much stronger. But then again, men generally have larger salaries; men generally have a lot more support; they don't have children.

There was a time where I was driving a car, probably back still in '87, and for no particular reason, I started to cry. It really, it was like an unexpected thundershower, just buckets and buckets of tears. I was thinking to myself, "Why am I crying? Why am I?" I knew that I had this illness and this illness was depression. I had always thought otherwise, but depression is very physical. I also realized that my body needed that depression, but at the same time, it shouldn't go on and on. That made me aware of the fact that there is going to be an awful lot that I've got to deal with, my health, not just physical illness, to me it's mental, emotional, spiritual and physical. Actually, physical is like one of the last things that you have to treat. Mental stability is very important, because you cannot live without mental stability. Emotional stability, you can't live without that. And the spiritual, determining for yourself who God is, or what God is.

Coming out

Yvonne Knuckles I was at the AIDS Walk on Sunday. WORLD had a table. This girl, she said, "Just look Bunny, you hardly see any Afro-American people here." They should have been there. We have the highest rate of positive people now, Afro-Americans. I don't know why but they won't come out. Black people have been pushed back so long so it's that fear. If I come out people think . . .

The women that I know that are HIV-positive, that have AIDS, they have a fear of being rejected and they don't like to talk about it. They won't tell it. They won't get treatment. Basically, they stay off into a shell they like to do stuff under. My best friend has AIDS and we used all those years together and I can use her for an example. I kept telling her. I said, "We need to test because we shared needles." She wouldn't test. About seven months ago she got really, really sick. She kept this cough. She kept getting pneumonia, I kept telling her, "You probably have HIV." Finally they tested her and now she has 117 T-cells; she's going blind; she can't hear and she still won't tell anyone.

When you're stressing, you're back sitting in the car. I wonder if this person looking at me, has someone else told her? Do you know I've got it? That's worse than telling it. You have to tell 'em, just come on out. But everyone is not strong like that. It's because of the ignorance that people still have fear. So why shouldn't you give people love? You gotta talk, it's the best education. For me, when I was told, I needed someone to tell me I wasn't dying. I needed someone with the virus to tell me I wasn't going to die.

Hearing about WORLD

Nancy Lemoins I got really sick. I went in the hospital the last day of 1992 and I was in the hospital for a month and a half and I was really sick almost the whole year of 1993. When I started getting well, I went on a WORLD retreat. That was my first experience with WORLD and it was just such a great experience. I actually was in this room with this other woman named Carol Darling. She really affected me because she was the first person who I knew I was pretty close friends with who died and I don't know. The retreat was so very wonderful and I just really liked WORLD. I started getting involved with WORLD. I started going to retreats when I got better and now I volunteer there and I do mailings and speak for them. Now, a lot of my friends I know from WORLD.

Hazel Betsey I got involved with WORLD 'cause I went on one of their retreats. That's when I started seeing women infected. It was like 100 women there and they were all infected. I was amazed. I thought, this is so much cool. I think the biggest trip for me was seeing the different types of women that are infected. I was sitting there with my mouth open because there was young girls, sixteen, seventeen who were infected.

The day of the retreat, I got my blood test back and I found out that I lost three T-cells. I was losing my mind. I went to the bus to go to the retreat and I was like, "Oh, I got my blood work back and I lost three T-cells." Then I started talking to this woman. She was like, "Three, you lost three T-cells? How many have you got now?" I said, "132." She said, (*laughs*) "I have seven and I have had seven for the last five years." And I said, "No fucking way." She said, "Way." 'Cause in my head, I know that if I had seven T-cells, I would be losing my fucking mind, but I was around all these women who were so strong who had no T-cells and so many less than me that had kids.

I thought, Damn, what if I had to drag a kid through my life? And they're doing it, women that have infected children, women that are grandmothers that are infected, these women that were infected by their husbands, gosh. I'm a black woman; I used drugs, that's why I got infected. I kind of lessened myself and then I saw these women and some of them were addicts and some of them weren't. What do we do now? Just wallow in it or just lay down and die? Or do we support each other? And that's what I got, support. And that's what I saw. And that's what every woman there needed.

Advice

Marija Mrdjenovic   Well, usually my advice to all women is to keep on fighting. The men do understand it, not the doctors, but the gay men who I know who have HIV? They know. They know what they have to do. And they are aware. I talk to them all the time and we're basically in accordance; we're in agreement. But for women I would say, "Don't give up." The biggest problem is just that the women are just obediently dying. And they shouldn't be so damn obedient. Not only women with HIV. I ran into a woman who's having disk operations. She was in a great deal of pain. We were both in the waiting room at an X-ray lab, and we started talking. I told her that she must keep fighting because there are answers coming down the way, very important answers. She mustn't think that everyone has given up on her, and she must remember to support herself on her family, make them support her. Even if they don't feel like supporting her, make them. Use them.

PART V

Body, Culture, and Spirit

Rev. Mark Stanger We're just short-sighted. When I was growing up we were all taking polio vaccine in the '50s. There's always some terror out there. The city is the place of culture and life and interaction and commerce and creativity, but there's always danger. There's always danger where people are huddled together in a mass, a crowd at a soccer game. When we were kids in Catholic School in the Midwest there was a terrible fire in a big school in Chicago. Many children died. Nuns died and nuns threw kids out windows to save their lives. That was held up to us as a lesson about being careful and about safety and about all the protection of that Catholic School atmosphere, yet danger was lurking even there (Cowan and Kuenster, 1996). And I think that's why the city of Florence, the city of San Francisco or anywhere, I mean, cities are wonderful places, it's the image we use for Heaven, City of God, the Heavenly Jerusalem. We don't talk about the great pasture. We talk about the city. It's been populated and built. But, like Venice it's built on canals, like here it's built on landfill and earthquake faults. That ambiguity exists. There's that ambiguity whether we have the plague or street crime. There are land mines and there are things to be tasted and savored everywhere and that's just what life is about. We try to sanitize it or we may see it as only dangerous and only menacing.

And having been here for the quake, we know that the image in the Midwest is that some day California is going to fall off into the sea. We don't feel that way here. We feel the main lines will fail and electricity will be off. Trucks won't get here with food and buildings will collapse. It won't be as quick and merciful as just falling into the sea. We know it's a lot more ambiguous and a lot more fraught with danger and uncertainty than something as pretty as that.

I guess I'm developing my own mythologies and my own feel for it here and why I ended up here. It has a sublime beauty here. We're this little island nation just perched, this gentle opening in the cliffs that Sir Francis Drake couldn't even see from his ship that opens into the great bay. It's this fragile little beautiful edge of a continent. And here we are . . .

FOURTEEN

AIDS and the American Psyche

"The whole planet lives under a death sentence," Rev. Mark Stanger argued. Interviewees tell stories about the tools they use to cope and adapt to the new reality. They demonstrate Bronfrenbrenner's (1979) point that human development involves the growing person learning to function within increasingly complex situations. Somehow we find ways to survive. Cohler (1989) explains that development, bolstered by resilience, flows like a river. If one tributary has dried up, it will flow down another. In relating coping strategies, interviewees make a case against determinism, demonstrating the uses of history and spirituality to take on disease.

Confrontations between morality, disease, sex, and religion unleash deeply imbedded questions within the American psyche. Interviewees plead for the country's institutions to look beyond "fake Victorian values" and attempt to confront this disease honestly. From Ronnie Ashley's forgiveness of those who have harmed him, to Rev. Stanger's battles with faith after a lifetime in a monastery, the specter of disease becomes intimately entangled within the age old meditation: how will I live?

Robin Tichane I think New York City culturally is about half-way between London and Paris, whereas the rest of the country is firmly rooted in North America. Outside of Manhattan, you realize we have cultural and religious values making us so different from Europe.

You know all of the more liberal religious thinkers stayed in Europe. It was the outcasts, the conservative crazies, the Pilgrims, the Puritans, the Quakers, all the people who were just fringe nobody could handle over there. They all came over here. That colored a lot of the development of this country, so we have lots of crazy thinkers. This country has attracted a slew of fringe folks; that mixture makes this country very different than, say, the Enlightenment and Europe.

Tichane (1993) has written extensively about his life and times. Tichane's writing melds into an inquiry and statement about America by sketching his own journey from Iowa to New York City to California. He writes about the late '60s San Francisco, the '70s Zen Centers, and Green Gulch, concluding, "Finally one discovers that the frontier is not the west, it is yourself, rather a fresh look at living and the compelling appeal of the virgin land." Tichane elaborated in our interview.

Coming out here, Oriental religions are more prevalent because, for one thing, it is just across this little puddle called the Pacific. Those ideas of being one with nature were very current in the Sierra Club but also it's very in tune with Chinese and Japanese philosophies. It was OK out here to get into Zen Buddhism. The appeal is realizing it's not only your environment, it's not the landscape itself that is challenging. It's looking inside yourself and finding, "Oh, this is the adventure." I feel kind of fortunate that by the time I was twenty-five I discovered that it wasn't physical locale that determines how you discover yourself, it's inside.

Ronnie Ashley and I sat in the back patio of Uncle Burnies, a bar on 18th and Castro, soaked in the warm sun outside, "So I can really smoke," Ronnie explained as he pulled a pipe and a bag of grass from the leather pouch. He laughed and reflected upon the extremes of etiquette he has confronted working in the San Francisco AIDS Industry. "I get cover letters saying, 'I'm culturally competent.' . . . How the fuck do you become culturally competent? I am Native American and not even I am culturally competent." With beads woven through his long braided hair cropped up on the sides, wearing Bermuda shorts and a button-up Hawaiian shirt, staring through his spectacles and grinning through his scruffy mustache, Ronnie Ashley, or Chaka, reconstructed his history of an intact self (Borden, 1992). He told me the story of his life from a childhood of prostitution and heroin and the coping involved as he moved from a reservation in Texas, to Alabama, up to Cornell Cooking School in Ithaca, New York before ending up in San Francisco. Ronnie's life becomes a case study in adaptation (Lazarous and Folkman, 1984; Bowlby, 1979; Elson, 1988; Levinson, 1978). "I'm on Indian time," he explains, optimistically reflecting the insight that his struggle is part of the history and makeup of a people who have already endured one genocide (McAdams, 1990).

On growing up here

Ronnie Ashley   I was born August the 3rd, 1953, on the Tiqua Indian Reservation which is in Isleta outside of El Paso, Texas, born and raised on the reservation, born addicted to heroin, born to junkie parents. I spent my youth in the streets of El Paso, on the farms, on the cotton fields. It was still against the law in Texas to teach Indians how to read. I got as far as the sixth grade. It wasn't until I got older that I got my GED [high school equivalency exam] and everything else. I was a child prostitute until I guess I was thirteen, when I got a train, hopped on over to Birmingham, Alabama which was an eye-opener to say the least. It was so funny because the oppression being on the reservation with the Missions and assuming that it was only us that were being discriminated against until I ended up in Birmingham, only to find out that they didn't like black people either.

Mom was only thirteen years old when she had me. She is only thirteen years older that I am. I am going to be forty-three years old. They had nine kids. Living on the reservation was like burnt mean and oppression. There was no running water. There was no electricity. The land that we had, we all grew our own vegetables and corn. The Rio Grande was our bathing water, our bathrooms; that was it.

The United States history, it's well known for its bad immigration laws. (*Laughs.*) The Mission and the Catholic Church were a big part of the reservation. We were forced into Catholic schools; we were shaved; we couldn't speak our own dialects. You are ostracized from your own community because you end up going into Catholic churches and having to abide by their rules and regulations. And by the time you went back to the reservation you'd lost the ability to speak your own language. You've converted to the white ways. It was double whammy.

They can strip you of your religion, your hair. They are able to strip you of your language, your clothes, but the soul of who you are as an individual and where you come from and are born with always stays with you regardless of the environment you are shoved into. For a long time, I did not understand why I was being treated the way I was being treated. I did not understand why I was a savage; I didn't understand why my native tongue couldn't be spoken or why I couldn't go to school.

In my stuff, as far as being a junkie and prostitution at such a young age, the fact was that that was my only outlet. There was nothing nice about the reservation. What the fuck did I want to stay there for? I knew how to work on the farms. I'd been there since I was two. Where do you go from there? That's why I just got on the train and headed out to Birmingham, Alabama. Why there? I don't know. That's beyond my belief, really. (*Chuckles.*) I ended up on the cotton fields out there and just started working, making some money.

Growing up in Birmingham, Alabama was probably the hardest thing that I ever did. But at the same time I think it was probably the biggest lesson. Working at Shanti Project we talk about multiculturalism and we talk about acceptance and diversity. The '60s taught me diversity; that gave me strength; that gave me hope. That, if anything else, still kept your dignity intact. It's not just one's pride, it's who you are as a human being. Here you have communities who are prejudiced against you because you are Indian or because you are black or because of your sexuality. Here you're Native American, you're gay, your lover is black. I always had the sense, you do unto others what is done unto you regardless of how ugly some stuff can be. Yet sometimes I would like to do unto others what is done unto me because sometimes it just fucking feels good. You can no longer just continuously turn the other cheek because it's convenient. I think my own history dictated that to me. I was always under the impression to form my own steps, my own history. This was how I saw the world.

It wasn't about being black or white or red or yellow or anything. The way that we were always taught, we're all God's people, regardless of what sand you're molded out of; we're all people of color. It's not just the black, the red, the yellow and the green as far as those who are the people of color. No, white people are still people of color and we should not forget that. It's just a matter of the different pieces of clay into which we are going to be molded. That's always been my thinking as far as people and life and how I was going to go about changing. It's kind of weird because my history was already written for me as an Indian, at least the hundreds of years prior.

History

My history, my own ancestry, it's blood and it's natural history of who we are as a people from this earth, our pottery, our clay. We are in it. We are buried in it. We are born in it. That is my history, that is who I know of who I am as this particular tribe and as this particular people and not "what is now the United States" and what they put out on history books for us to learn who we are. You have tribes that are acknowledged by the United States and you have those that are not. If the United States were to turn around to correct a wrong into a right, feasibly it can't. It can acknowledge the fact that this is who we are but otherwise, it's like to turn around and tell the millions of people and New York and these other cities, "Excuse me, it's time that you are going to have to leave." You just can't give back what was taken from people hundreds of years ago. It's real hard to correct the actions.

There's a lot of history here for all people that we have to acknowledge, but yet at the same time we can't continue to beat a dead horse. I am sorry what the Europeans, the Spaniards and the French did to my people. I am also sorry what my people did to them during the time of war. I can't change that, but we can turn around and acknowledge the atrocities and then see how we can move forward, take that ugliness and pick out the constructive part, the positive attitude about that ugliness and move people forward on that same level. We can't continue with all this anger and hatred with people because of their race or sexuality or whatever the fucking situation may be, or else we aren't ever going to get nowhere. Either we embrace everyone as all and as one or we embrace no one.

Growing up in the '60s, there was all the riots and stuff that were going down in the Black Hills and the Pine Ridge Reservation, the manhunt for Leonard Peletier, the burning down of the Federal Building and all this shit that the American Indian Movement was doing at the time, trying to get the United States to recognize the crap as far as the Sioux under the jurisdiction of the Pine Ridge Reservation and the Black Hills and wanting to have the monument blown up. Vietnam was happening. Nixon was going on. You had all this crap going down in the United States, including everything in Birmingham in the '60s all the way up until the early '70s with segregation going down in Boston as well. That was still part of the climate, still part of who the United States were and their understanding of who we were as a people.

Marija Mrdjenovic I have a theory that you are a composite of all your ancestors, that they are still within you. When I was in the hospital in '90, my fevers were 104, going up to 105 sometimes, a little higher. Then I'd go through these racking body chills where you could put a million blankets on me and I'd still be freezing. I just got so tired of it that one night I called on all my ancestors and I said, "Please, come to me now." I called on my family; I called on everyone. I said, "If you can hear me, please help me now." I went back as many generations as I could, possibly, to ask them to please help me now. Next day, I was just fine. I was relaxed. I was calm. I was healthy. I was ready to get the hell out of there. The doctor was taken aback; he thought, "Maybe she'll have a relapse or something." And I didn't. I learned that that is there, that is the strength that is available to me.

I think for Native Americans the strength of your ancestors is in you. I think that a lot of that has been lost in modern medicine, has been thrown out as too primitive. An important part of healing is where you find your strength, where you find that. I don't really see God as God. I see nature as a strong force in my life; I see history as a very strong force in my life. I'll talk to whatever I think God is, but I really find more that I feel like I'm talking to my ancestors.

Hank Wilson Personally, I went and read all the Holocaust books I could when the epidemic started. I went to the Jewish Community Center and I read every autobiography about somebody who survived the Holocaust. And I think there'll be some people who'll survive. I also think we know that there's a lot of people who won't.

In November 1994, the Church of the Advent in San Francisco held AIDS Day at the Advent services. Fr. Mark Stanger gave a sermon on "The Stages of AIDS Anger." I hadn't even known he was positive. The following week I contacted him and he got back to me immediately. He arrived at my apartment dressed no differently than any other urbanites in the city, in black cut-off jean shorts rolled up above the knee, a T-shirt, buzzed hair, black sneakers, an earring. Over coffee that sunny morning, Fr. Mark told me the story of his life from a childhood outside Chicago in the '50s through entering a Benedictine monastery when he was twenty-one, where he was ordained a Roman Catholic priest and stayed for the following fourteen years. "It was one of the most important periods of my life. In some ways I'll never recover from the good and the bad that I experienced while I was there. It really was formative." In Italy, where he was also conducting research on original sources for his doctoral work, he found himself in a power struggle with the abbot. In 1986, he left the order and moved to Minneapolis, no credit, no work history. One more change was in store. "As I was getting settled there in September, I went for an HIV test and I found out that I was positive. That really set me into a tailspin because I was going just to reassure myself that I wasn't," Mark recalled. The following is Fr. Mark's story of relearning how to live in the city of man, reconciling disease, the past, faith and life in Baghdad by the Bay.

Mark Stanger People ask whether I left Benedictine life because of being gay and maybe it had to do with that. Really it had to do with authority. Being gay is one of the reasons I would never go back, but I didn't see that as my major difficulty.

Parting glances, out to San Francisco

Before that was little crushes in the monastery and secret things, but you couldn't meet people the way people do all throughout their twenties. It was kind of fun. After many false starts, I met someone who was twelve years my junior. It was interesting because I had actually lost a dozen years. He was just beginning to make plans to move to San Francisco. Now, as I told people then, I had been lots of places, lived in Italy, in Germany, two extended trips to Israel. I had been camping on the Gaza Strip but I had never been west of the Rockies. I had never had a mythology about San Francisco. I didn't even know about California geography. I had never read *Tales of the City*. It just didn't interest me, but this guy did interest me. So I moved out here.

Being from the New World and coming to the Old World, that's like meeting your grandfather. It's really difficult, like you can't get in. My psychiatrist was very good. She helped me integrate Old World culture into my own. And going to the Mideast helped me deal with Christian roots and something more primitive and symbolic, not Cartesian Western logical linear but circular and deep, and archaeological sites and layers, symbolic activity, Islam, Judaism, Christian roots; it's the Mediterranean world where people don't have to prove anything. They live, young Italian guys, they just stand in the Piazza in the afternoon. They don't have to, they just are. They have all the millennia of history reeking out of them. They're not uncomfortable. They just know how to do it. They don't have to go to cooking school or go to William Sonoma. They have all that stuff. And we're still learning. We're just on the frontier. We're just cowboys out here and American culture has some wonderful things but it's still being born.

Re-entering the Church

It's very interesting that I revived my religious life in San Francisco. My two years in Minneapolis I couldn't go into a church. I would get too angry. It was a person with AIDS, another former monk who brought me to Church of the Advent. He's dead now, Geary Gerard, and he said, "You might be interested in this." And I said, "Well, I might come here to worship but I'm going to remain anonymous," and I got involved. A whole part of me was restored that I thought I wouldn't have again. I got to teach theology at the school for deacons. It turned out to be wonderful and to be openly gay and have a bishop who gave me a chance and to go through a process of testing for three years before they listed me as a priest, that was frustrating, but I did it.

Sex and shame and learning to live

Now to say something else about the stigma, I'm ashamed. I'm not proud of the sexual experiences I had during the fourteen years where I was supposed to be living celibate. I can say as much as I want in my defense. I lived that life, the religious life with all its traditional expectations, pretty well for fourteen years. I could have gotten in a lot more trouble than I did. The fact is, that is when I did become infected, probably during my European sojourn when I was going through a particularly tough time and did some crazy things. So I think I've had the virus since, I have reason to believe, August of 1982. I don't think any of us have to apologize for our sexual experiences. I think sex is just sex. But when you are committed either to not have sex or to have sex with only certain people and you're breaking that commitment, I think that's serious. There's a certain dishonesty and so I'm not proud of that, but I have a souvenir to remind me. I wanted to be the perfect monk. It's kind of a spiritual pride, a kind of narcissism I guess.

By the way, both the men, the man I am in a relationship with now and my former, are negative. That amazes me. I mentioned that in the sermon two weeks ago. People can analyze why other people do this or that but it's just one more bit of evidence that people with HIV need to get on with their lives, whatever they're doing, their work, their interests, their play, their loving, whatever it is, and just keep going.

Sister Death or a rip-off?

I think in general I have made peace with the virus although it still denotes loss of function and deterioration and death. That's inescapable. Maybe I do believe in the Christmas soccer game (in which English and German soldiers played Christmas Day soccer game on the front during WW I). When I go away for the weekend, I'm not going to even pack the AZT. But I never really forget about it. I don't have this worked out yet, what my relationship is to the virus inside, whether I'm at war and at odds with it or whether I've made my peace or it's somewhere in the middle. Maybe I have these temporary truces? And then other times I get pissed off and just want to get rid of it.

There will be, I hope, there will be a moment where I embrace Sister Death, I hope, but not now. I'm not in the business of dying now. Even though we keep death daily before our eyes and we're all mortals and all flesh is grass and all. That is true. But right now I am alive and I'm about the business of living. I haven't even begun to learn how to exercise all my creativity and energy into doing that.

No, I don't see a sword of Damocles. It's more like the time bomb in a way. It sounds crass, but I remember as a kid, a line from the Stations of the Cross about the Ignominious Death on the Cross. Part of our myth that talks about an ignominious death. Regrettably, Christianity has been reduced to moral teaching. People have watered down the myths and the rituals. Mystery religion is a part of Christianity. Christianity promises contact, incorporation with the Divine. That is so attractive and yet so frightening that we usually sanitize it. I don't think it has something special for PWAs, it has something special for people who are disposed that way, a chance to enter into this history and myth and for it to become real, to say I want to become part of this divine story. I want to eat and drink at this place where the divine doesn't judge but welcomes. I want to be part of something that gives me reassurance in the service oriented parts of my life.

Spirituality, fundamentalism and roadblocks to prevention

Dan Vojir   I was Catholic in a very formal religion. The fact is, I have a gut feeling that there is a God. Now my only spirituality would be, "For God's sake! Why in the hell did you do this to me?" That's spirituality too, no matter what anybody says. There's the other side of trying to help other people. That's more spiritual than anything else, I think.

I have a real ingrained feeling about the fundamentalist right from what I have read of the actual Bible and the way I was brought up. I simply will state that I think these people are idiots. Anybody who takes a King James Bible and says that every word is absolute is just a moron. The Bible went through so many different translations before it ever went English. In the translation from Greek alone, some words would have ten different meanings. I can understand why they say God just intended everything to just come out exactly the way it did. I can understand why they would say it, but that's not true.

One of my authors, Dan Helminak, who's the author of the book *What the Bible Really Says About Homosexuality* (1994). He's a Roman Catholic theologian, a very good guy, and I placed him on a radio station along with Fred Phelps. I called Dan the other night and said "How did it go?" He says, "I enjoyed it." Phelps, by the way, stalked out after twenty minutes and Helminak carried on the whole hour. This guy said something about where in the Bible it said, "He shall take the faggots, put the faggots into the fire." Dan caught him off guard. He says, "Really? Where is that quote? I hadn't seen that. That's great!" He said, first of all, there's never been a quote like that. Secondly, if it were faggots, it would have meant bundles of sticks of wood and thirdly, it was probably a translation for poker. And Phelps is running for governor of Missouri.

Remember what I told you, when we had our first theology class in high school, the priest looked us straight in the eye and said, "The nuns were very, very nice ladies for sure. Forget everything they ever taught you about religion. We're starting from day one." We learned, don't believe "that Methusela was 956 years old! All they wanted to tell ya was that he was a wise man. That's all. They equated age with wisdom so they said he was 956 years old. If one shepherd says he's got thousands and thousands of sheep, it merely means that he had five more than the guy next door to him." And we're supposed to go to the Bible and believe every single comma and every single dot, every single paragraph and every single phrase? "The Lord's Prayer," you know, the only words he probably did say were "Our Father." For hundreds of years, scholars have been trying to tell people, take the Bible in context.

I was thinking about something the other day. Because of this new right-wing backlash, I would love to be able to get back at them where it hurts. Maybe a final absolute reaction of all the theologians in the world and just saying, "Stop the crap already." And putting it into like an annotated Bible that would become, hopefully, an incredible best seller that everybody would be reading and be incredibly influenced by it. I would love to see that happen. A lot of this is a "religious war."

Right-wing Christians are the ones who basically broke away from the traditional teachings. These were much more lenient, much less "the Bible says this word for word." Fundamentalists were the heretics. With this book I am proposing, you would find a movement that would just be so back against Christian fundamentalism, that it would, hopefully, counteract any homophobia and AIDS phobia and things like that.

Beyond fake Victorian values

Mark Stanger I'm going to raise the name of a failure, Christine Gebby. The beginning of her undoing was when she said, "We have got to get rid of these fake Victorian values about sex." I absolutely think that's number one and that's under education/prevention. It means talking about sex all the time to young people and it just has to be done. Even J. Everett Coop, this ridiculous Baptist whatever he was, he went to Ronald Reagan and he said, "Look, we have to get real sex education and real prevention. We have to do it."

Cynora Jones The churches need to confront it. They really do. I was over in Engleside in San Francisco. I went into the church and told him I was working in the neighborhood and I'd be glad to maybe come and do an AIDS 101. He said, "Oh, we don't have a problem with that; we teach abstinence," and shooed me out. OK, I come out and there are some girls, like thirteen with their Catholic little uniforms and there's a group of guys. I walk over and ask them if they would like some condoms. Those very girls were like, "Oh yeah, give us some! Give me some!" But he ran me out because his head is up his ass, thinking "These kids are abstaining." So what do you tell them when somebody dies in church from AIDS? What do you tell them when priests are getting diagnosed?

FIFTEEN

Battle Cries, AIDS, and the Arts

Arts communities have been devastated by AIDS (Fong-Torres, 1993). This loss has metamorphosed into a dynamic progression in the arts in San Francisco. Art work produced in San Francisco by visual artists with AIDS covers an impressively wide emotional and intellectual territory, bringing into its multifold range themes of hardship, community, reification, autonomy, separateness and liberation. The work of the San Francisco positive art movement allows members to reconcile themselves with irrevocable pasts, losses, and joys of previous eras through catharsis. Marcuse (1977: 73) suggests that "remembrance of things past would become a mode of struggle for changing the world." Whether or not the work possesses a style all its own is for academics to debate. But one thing is certain, most of this art is strong enough in content and in form to constitute a movement all its own. Per recalls the first wave of artists he knew who were hit by the plague and what happened to their worlds.

Per Eidspjeld The fact that all these wonderful things were going on – that got my admiration for the Bay Area. I went to lots of art openings and museums; here were all these cute little galleries and parties and flowers and wonderful stuff. Working artists lived here and other queens and friends would cater to make wonderful events happen.

Of course when AIDS came around, many of these artists were some of the first people to get sick. So, of course, the people who were making all the food, the flowers and all the arrangements were the first in line to care for these people. There was all this hysteria: don't touch, and use rubbers and gloves. The police were wearing gas masks. They had the riot gear. That was the end of many of the parties.

It created big holes in the whole arts communities; creative people who were established and all of a sudden they were just taken away from this place. So it changed the face of art. The art that followed sort of gives you a portrait of what's going on in this city. You can look at art and you can sort of go: What's going on here? Who are these people? So it became very dark and kind of like the music scene. I don't like the music through the '80s but I went out dancing anyway. And then the '70s came back and I feel so happy. (*"Then the '80s came back," I add.*) I think we should get past the '80s. It's the '90s now and let's get real. Let's get smart. Time to wake up.

Battle Cries, the Visual AIDS Show

Spring 1995, the smokers stood in the yard outside the warehouse on Alabama Street at "Battle Cries," a show of work by Visual AIDS artists. Nancy was inside, Robin Tichane's work also showed inside. Several hundred people came to the show, a large number for a local showing. Outside, Marcos Reyes shared a Marlboro Red with me. He wore jeans, a long overcoat, wire-rim glasses, a yellow scarf wrapped around his neck, and a group of colorful pins on his jacket proclaiming respectively, "I've Got a Huge Dick!" "I'm Illegal!" and "I'm Positive."

"Well that's all we need to know now, isn't it?" I commented.

Our interview continued with the question of the function of private information serving as public protest. Marcos explained that the process of being told he could no longer receive services because he was illegal, due to Proposition 187, illustrated that he did not exist; being told that he was gay and was going to die told him that his voice did not exist. After that period of cultural/personal flattening, Marcos came out. He talked about the process of finding his voice again as a triple "other": illegal, gay, and HIV-positive. As we drank coffee at Muddy Waters at the corner of 16th and Mission, Marcos explained that the social construct built around HIV is even more painful than the physical ramifications of the disease itself. Through expression he found his way out of the No Exit.

Marcos Reyes I'm discovering I got a really bad identity crisis right after I move up here. I got to this point where I didn't know who the hell I was. While living in L.A., I did everything you can imagine until finally I landed in this place in a pet supply store where I worked for four years. It was a survival I guess. I didn't mind. I had to pay my bills like everybody else and I wanted to get somewhere. But it was more difficult than I thought. I don't think it was the city by itself. I was getting sicker and I started public assistance and I was humiliated. I didn't want to do it. The problem with AIDS I think is the very slow progression of symptoms, and in order for you to survive, at least at this time, you have to invest more time in your health. When I applied for those services, I felt like I had failed. After all, I don't have control of my life and you are witnessing, for once, the decay. How long it will take I don't know, but it's a social illness after all too.

Here is another thing, now all this business related to Proposition 187 blah, blah, blah, it's like they are bringing all these images on TV about immigrants being criminals. You wonder where all these people came with all those ideas and how much the general population believes them. So that's another issue that we had to fight. It's like, I'm not a criminal. I'm a very productive person. You have to explain this a lot to yourself because at that point you think, Is that really my image?

Sometimes it's just like a double stigma or three times the stigma. You are from another ethnic group, you have a contagious disease, and you have another sexual preference. Those are aspects that define my person. I discovered after this identity crisis I had a year ago that I didn't have any voice. I was losing control again of my life. I was getting sicker and I thought I was at the "No Exit" point. I was stuck. All my motivation was gone. I was getting angry and tired of people. Fighting these stereotypes can be very draining sometimes.

One time I was in college. I was in one of my classes and I was with a group of people talking. This woman was asking this guy about fixing something in her house, some kind of gardening work or construction work. I was just listening. She looks at me and she asks me, "Do you want to do this job?" I told her, "No, I don't know how to do that. I never done it before." Then she looks at me like, "So how do you do for a living." And I went just red because for the first time, I felt like she sees my face and she expects that I should be cleaning houses. She doesn't imagine that I have a degree in psychology. She doesn't imagine that I'm a manager in a business place. The other one is when people ask me if I like burritos and they say, "Well you're Mexican aren't you?" And I say, "Yeah, but we don't have burritos in Mexico City." See, you have to explain yourself in many aspects.

I was in this point of no exit and I didn't know where to go. One time I discovered myself crying because I didn't know who the hell I was. I wasn't the professional that left Mexico, 'cause I haven't done this in a long time. I wasn't a photographer because I didn't feel like creating anything. I didn't want to be the manager of a pet store. I felt like my dreams were some place else. But then I kept telling me, well I have to take responsibility for all my choices. The way I rescued this, which I believe is like a self-esteem issue, is to talk about this.

When you saw me with my pics at the art show, I discovered that I was actually a public figure. I realized that I was doing a job. It was not just that I have two pictures on the wall, but the fact that I was there and that people wanted to talk with me. I discovered that voice again, a very badly needed voice. I guess the more you are portrayed as something that you don't identify with, the more you want to. You have to let people know it's not this way. It doesn't work that way. I decided to use that voice in my photography.

In addition to being a wonderful storyteller, Robin Tichane stands as one of the city's new generation of artists. Tichane's work offers new paradigms with which to consider the world of AIDS. As a participant in the Students for a Democratic Society and the Anti-War Movement before he got involved in the Gay Liberation Movement of the '70s, elements of the battle for personal freedom were not unfamiliar to him, especially as San Francisco began to feel like a city under siege by AIDS in the early '80s. Liberation takes many forms in Tichane's work. His 1994 show "AIDS Into Art: A Look In, Not At!" exhibited at three San Francisco locations over three months. The show incorporated his suite of wood block prints entitled "AIDS' Dark Terrain: Twelve Stations from a Yankee Pilgrim." The twelve prints, each a horizon of sorts, serve as allegories for internal and external panoramas. In Tichane's world, physical terrains meld into psychological landscapes. I asked him about his formidable task of "creating a visual equivalent to the emotional response to HIV infection."

Robin Tichane Oh, I get goose bumps, see (*showing me his arm*). To me it's very exciting. I feel very fortunate, I've had enough time in friends who have died and my buddy who died and my own diagnosis to kind of stand back and begin to develop a little perspective. Because of my conservation work I'm used to projecting into past eras and back into say early nineteenth-century American transcendental landscapes or medieval icons and to try to envision different cultures. But it takes perspective to begin to kind of realize where the elements of that are. By retiring when I did, I've had enough time to begin to have some perspective on what is happening today and in the near future.

Engaged art

Nancy Lemoins I don't know what people do understand about this. I do understand that there is a lot of denial in terms of women. I think women are still kind of in that "I can't get it" stage, especially sexually. I can't say anything that everybody hasn't said a thousand times. In fact, the painting I'm doing right now is, "It Could Have Been You." I'm not any different. It's so funny, it's just exactly like this painting which also says, "Look through what separates us." People do that enough; they look at me and go, "She was this and that's why it couldn't be me." I'm pretty poor so I use my Rainbow Card and my Visual AID stuff. I get a lot of that attitude from people. I just want to say, "Fuck you." I used to be intimidated by that and now I'm just very angry and kind of militant. I just won't take that attitude at all.

I really came to this realization that I know I'm going to die of this. I used to think that maybe I wasn't, but I know I will. I don't know how soon it's going to be, but in fifty years or twenty years or however many years when there's a cure and this is all over and it's some little footnote in a history book, I want there to be something that names people and feelings and emotions and is a really personal vision. Art is the best historian; it's the most personal historian. That's why I do what I do.

Everything I do is HIV-related now. I had a really hard time with that for a long time. I don't know if I want to be so overt and use words like "It could have been you" in a painting. But I just gave into it and it's OK. I actually had an opening at this HIV showing on Sunday. You know, the companion piece to the "I'll not go gently" one. This woman was sobbing. It's what every artist wants. She was like, "This is so great. This is it. You're saying what I want to hear." That's what makes me keep painting because I certainly don't sell paintings. I know that people really like my stuff, but they don't want that much HIV in their living room. It's hard for people and I respect that.

Representations of AIDS

Robin Tichane A lot of the images of AIDS that are current, if not trendy, say from the '80s almost through to today, are black and white photographs of people with AIDS. That's what I think the general public associates with art about AIDS. In addition, they very often are by artists who do not have an AIDS diagnosis and they are not caring for a person with AIDS. Many of them are professional photographers who go in and take very close-up snapshots of faces. They are kind of big blown-up heads and confrontational and horrific. I find them very disturbing. I think they are taking advantage of a bruised group of people. It's very voyeuristic and it's not benefiting the people who are being photographed. It's book publishers making money from the publication of these books. By having their things in both the Museum of Modern Art Portrait Collection and the Museum of Black and White Photographers, they are making a buck out of it, whereas there are some gay artists who, say, have lovers who are dying of AIDS and they take photographs of them. There's a sympathetic non-confrontational look. I am very offended by a lot of that looking "at." It's a journalistic approach the broadcast media and the print media use to sell television and newspapers. Even the AIDS Foundation has hired Annie Lebowitz, paid hard cash to her, to take these photographs and I am just appalled.

I had already been working on the thrust of my work, being a little more understated in the dark planes before I was too explicit about the subject matter. It was an interior look. I think one of the difficult things about AIDS is the look of the disease, which frightens and scares most people. You know the lesions and the gaunt look and the pneumonia complications. I think people do have an inner life. When people become so sick, they go look at themselves in the mirror in the bathroom and they have a lot less esteem simply because of the way they look, but their inner life is still them and that's their core. I think people have to make a real effort to get beyond the look of AIDS and to think about the value of people inside. So that's what I mean when I say "AIDS Into Art: A Look In, Not At."

A reason to paint

Robert Boulanget AIDS has definitely given me permission to paint. You don't need that. Some people would say why do you need permission. Not all of us are all alike. We're all here to learn things. I think I discovered my creative energy and that was Tom. I truly believe I inherited a lot of that. I look at things and I see paintings everywhere and I sort of frame everything. It's really weird. It started after Tom died. I saw beauty everywhere.

SIXTEEN

Medications for Deviance

The story of the events precipitating today's evolving relationship between doctors and patients plays a dynamic role within this history. Many of the epidemic's greatest heroes were doctors. Others were uncomfortable working with a new disease in which little was known, the clues around which suggested it was acquired through deviant means. Although some PWAs have very good relationships with their doctors, others had traumatic relationships. These are the stories of AZT, toxicity, cultural arrogance, and unintended abuse of authority in a place where all too often medicine is the only god.

A review of the underlying power dynamics within the social structure puts the doctor/patient relationship into context. According to Parsons (1951: 429–30), within the authoritarian doctrine of the doctor/patient relationship, the doctor and the patient have traditionally followed strictly delineated roles. Meyer and Rowan (1977: 22) explain that this frame forms rigid social obligations and expectations for both the doctor and the patient. The doctor, the trained medical professional, is entrusted with responsibility to manage the illness of the patient. The role of the patient is to accept passively the advice, expertise, treatment, and therapy of the doctor (Parsons, 1951: 429–30). This structure proved painfully ineffective when applied to treatment of the new affliction.

No news and good advice

In the early years of the AIDS epidemic, there was no form of treatment. Doctors had to admit they knew absolutely nothing, something doctors are not very good at. Doctors are trained to present their information with the full power of medical authority. So they presented what little information they had, that AIDS appeared terminal, as absolute fact. "You are going to die within a year," doctors told patient after patient, with traumatic consequences.

Parsons (1951: 429–30) makes clear that the problem of health is intimately involved within the functional necessities of the social system. Health is a prerequisite of the productivity. Lack of health is perceived as dysfunctional; it prevents the individual from fulfilling his or her social obligations to be a productive citizen. To the extent that health is controllable through responsible behavior, there is a functional interest for the society to control and minimize illness. Illness stems from laziness. Exposure to illness is perceived as motivated, the result of unconscious wishes to be injured so as not to have to play out the traditional expectation of work. For these reasons people bring about sickness themselves. Traditional morality explains many of the public health policies taken and not taken around the AIDS epidemic (Murray and Payne, 1988: 13; Bersani, 1988: 197; Rofes, 1996: 115).

Murray and Payne (1988: 13) argue that without a medical fix for HIV, medical practitioners blamed PWAs for their non-compliance with bourgeois mores. Consciously or unconsciously, medical professionals condemned their ill patients for their perceived deviations from normal behavior and lack of adherence to conventional lifestyles. The obligation to legitimate their prestige and authority created a pressure for the medical establishment to do something about the epidemic although the needs of the patients were often not taken into account.

In November 1995, the Journal of the American Medical Association published a significant study showing that doctors regularly ignore or misunderstand the requests of terminally ill patients (Gilbert, 1995; SUPPORT, 1995). Reports of doctors' refusals to follow patient directives have become a regular occurrence (Lewin, 1996). The following are the reactions of people whose wishes and complaints about the side effects and documented "limited usefulness" of new medications were neglected (Reuters, August 1995). These specific views about treatment are not presented as facts; I do not vouch for accuracy of the events in these stories. However, the bewilderment and negative views of the medical establishment are also facts. This chapter allows interviewees to tell stories about a profession which makes a habit of ignoring their voices. Here are the voices behind these reports. For those mistreated, too often their pain, their confusion, and their wisdom have not been heard.

Marija Mrdjenovic When I have observational researchers look at me, they are not looking at me, they are looking at my illnesses. One of the arguments that you hear all the time is that, "Well, it might help the HIV." So let it! You know? (*Laughs.*) As long as it helps me, my body might be able to better fight the HIV. But the attitude of a lot of the doctors is, "I am God. I alone can save you; I can come up with a cure." It's that

Superman image. Unfortunately, the only thing that can really cure anyone is their own body and that is totally overlooked.

Modern medicine is the military. From the Civil War on, every hospital was designed to use the military approach to solving illness, finding the magic bullet; being that conquering general prevailed. You can't order the body to heal; you've got to help it.

Ronnie Ashley Now, people are all of a sudden using "Alternative Medicine!" They are using traditional Native American herb rituals, using Chinese acupuncture and pressures and herbs and medicines. Here is medicine that has been with us for thousands of years and now all of a sudden it's "alternative therapy." The scientists around the United States and the people around the world are finally honoring it.

Cautionary tales, part one – prognoses of death

Jay, Brad, Cynora, Philip, Hazel, and Art among other interviewees were given life expectancies by their doctors. They tell similar stories.

Jay Segal The day you got your results back is sort of blown away. I did the normal HIV cocoon where you just hide. You take a lot of showers 'cause you feel dirty, major depression. Also back then, and still today, doctors are totally stupid, somehow think they're Gods; they give you life expectancies. Doctors cannot give a life expectancy. God does. And that is wrong because the thing that destroys the most T-cells the fastest is stress. Depression is stress.

Brad Sherbert My doctor gave me an AIDS diagnosis because I had thrush down to my lungs. I don't know about now, but back in '88 when you had thrush that goes all the way down to the esophagus, they gave you a terminal prognosis 'cause they said they couldn't stop it. And they told me I'd be dead in six months.

Philip Blazer Back in '87 I made these trips back and forth to Sacramento trying to get involved with this drug trial that Jonas Salk was developing. At the time, it was something they were going to come out with in months and they were getting volunteers. And they made it very clear that if your T-cells were under a certain level, they couldn't use you because you were going to be dead in a year. Point blank, that's what they said to this whole crowd of people at Davis. Well mine was below this certain level and they called me up at work to tell me this. You need to start taking this and this and this, this whole list of stuff. And I flipped. I remember running down the stairs of my building downtown and buying all these overpriced vitamins at one of these smoke shops in the high-rise. I was panicking. That was in '87. So I guess they didn't know what they were talking about.

Ugly memories – warning: toxic materials

John Cailleau   There was one guy I knew with HIV who looked like a Pillsbury Doughboy because he was taking vitamin C infusions doctors were advocating. This guy had to get hooked up to the usual IV bag at least once a day during the retreat so he could get his vitamin C, end up with this puffy moon face. That was pretty much a guinea pig situation.

Darnell Davis   When my lover started the radiation treatments, his doctor says, "Oh, you just have a little hair fall out and that's it." This man, he lived on the pride of his hair. All his hair fell out. Then he said they said it would clear up for the KS lesions and it did not clear up. Finally, close to the end he says, "Baby, will you be mad at me if I stop?" I says "No. If you want to stop, you stop; I'm behind you 100 percent."

A lot of people are taking things that are making them ill. I met a guy the other day that's taking Septra. And some people just can't take it. His doctor says, "Well, break it in quarters and take it." If your body don't want it, don't fucking put it in it. If your body's rejecting it, the doctor should never have convinced him to take it. Listen to your body. Doctors take this thing too lightly. Too many doctors do not educate themselves on what's going on.

Cynora Jones   I got diagnosed at this clinic with HIV so they directed me to the AIDS clinic in L.A. and I didn't really know which, I knew AIDS? HIV? what? It's still not really clicking, OK? I don't know if I can tell you this. (*Tears flow.*) So once I got there, oh God this is really . . ., they put me in a fucking sterile room with fifty other people and they're talking over our God damn heads! I don't know why I'm there! What am I doing? The doctor they put me in the room with, I'm sitting there in this clinical space and he comes in and tells me, "You have AIDS." I don't know his fucking name! Do you know what I'm saying!?! I get angry about this, still. I'm sitting there and I start crying. He says, "Save your tears, you're going to need your strength for the disease," and walked out. OK, I have been stigmatized in thirty seconds, OK?

Initial treatments

Art   If people believe there is nothing then they'll take what comes, and there is money. And doctors are scared, another thing they often won't cop to. If a doctor is scared, bases will be covered even if it's something he knows nothing about. Present it with some semblance of certainty, "This is good for you" when they don't know; and patients will listen 'cause they don't know. "I'll do what my doctor tells me."

Jay Segal   Treatment, I'm skeptical. I have been in several studies including 016 which was the first AZT study. It killed my two best friends within a month, AZT-related liver toxic disease. They were alcoholics. You can't drink and do AZT at the same time. But the only way to get these drugs now is in the studies because if you wait for them to be approved, you'll be dead. You gotta play their games.

Mark Stanger   I started taking AZT about six years ago. Eight years ago it was twelve capsules a day, people were running around with beepers. There was even something on the national news about the new San Francisco Mantra, you're in the subway or anywhere and you can hear beepers going off. There were two schools then. There were people who felt or intuitively hoped that AZT was some life-giving drug that every four hours gets into your body, and those who rejected it because it was the only one the government approved. And it wasn't all that effective. I was one of these people who like a good little monk, I set my clock at 3:00 a.m., wake up, pop two pills and I would fall right to sleep. Now I'm happy taking four to six tablets a day.

Philip Blazer   I took it for about four years, I have not taken it for a long time. The only problem I had with it was the alarm going off in the middle of the night, that alarm going off and having to reach for a bottle of AZT. I would wake up the next day and find a pile of AZT I had spilled all over the floor. The doctor told me later that I didn't have to take it in the middle of the night.

Jay Segal   When I started the AZT, they were extremely stupid back then. They gave 2400 milligrams a day. Now they give 300. It's a very toxic drug. But it's the most effective drug that we've come up with (*as of 1994*). It's had the most benefits, the most years of life, the most years of quality life than all other quality drugs combined and everybody hates it. Yucky side effects on it. It causes anemia in a lot of people. It causes fatigue from the anemia. It causes muscle wasting; you lose your butt. You have to go to the gym to put on muscles all the time because the disease and the drugs all eat the muscles.

AZT is a good drug. It got a lot of bad press lately. It doesn't work on everybody. It only works for X amount of time and X is different in everybody. But it does work. People should at least try it. If it works for you, wonderful, congratulations, you're a miracle baby. If it doesn't work for you try another one. The list goes on forever.

The idea of taking anti-retrovirals is to prolong your life and wait and stall and wait for the cure to come along. The cure's not going to come along, so that theory is completely debunked. But you can get a couple of really quality years of life.

Paul Greenbaum When I first started, AZT hadn't even been approved. It was actually approved for all the people under 200 T-cells the week that I was diagnosed. Thankfully that's not the way they do it now. It is a potent anti-viral for a year or so, but like I said I had high T-cells. I was taking AZT in combination with D4T even when my T-cells were a few hundred and I think maintaining a part of it. But there is a time after you become intolerant of it and that happened to me. Only we didn't know too much back in '89 or '90 about AZT and tolerance because people hadn't been taking it long enough. They either became intolerant of it with the first pill they took or they were successful at taking it. No one thought that after a year or two years that you could develop a tolerance but I became intolerant. I endured for several months continuing to take it before we kind of put it all together. I don't think it did any permanent damage but I must say I could sense a toxicity in my body.

Cautionary tales, part two

"If you don't take AZT I'm going to stop seeing you as your doctor," Gabriel, Hazel, and Marija were all informed by their doctors. Other doctors merely ignored complaints about side effects.

Marija Mrdjenovic At one point everyone wanted me to take AZT, i.e. "You have to take AZT." Well, I had had a very dear friend, who had AIDS, and had died after he'd been given 1200 milligrams of AZT. A complete overdose. At that time, as is now the case, the drug companies always go to the high end when they're testing their drugs. There have been so many people who have died of drug overdoses in clinical trials. You apply that to women and not only are they lower in body weight, they have a whole different immune system. You're giving them something that is even more than an overdose, it's an over-overdose.

One doctor wanted me to take these huge amounts of AZT and I refused. He said, "Well, if you don't take AZT I'm going to stop seeing you as your doctor." There was that attitude of, "I know what's best for you." I was convinced that AZT was not the answer. They wanted me to take like 600 to 800 milligrams and nowadays the optimum dosage is something like 300 to 600. They're still trying to push it up so they can sell more of the drugs, but literally, 300 was enough to give me arthritic symptoms and enough to bring my white cell count down.

Nancy Lemoins I took AZT for about three days once and then I threw the bottle out my kitchen window. That was like when it cost so much money. It just made me throw up constantly. I was much healthier. I had about 700 T-cells so it didn't even seem imminent.

At that meeting last night all the women had taken it for like a week and then they quit. Where all the men were like, yeah, I've been on AZT for forty-seven years.

Philip Blazer Then I just started feeling like I was getting toxic. I was having light skin problems that could have been the result of something else. And I cut my dosage in half. I went from 1200 to 600 milligrams. Within two weeks, the CDC recommended that people halve their dosages. Then came information about the body becoming immune to it after a while and not being able to fight back, it losing its effectiveness. I haven't really taken AZT for four years.

Hazel Betsey Back then there was like all this talk about how doctors are putting people on medication right away when they are first diagnosed. They were treating them like guinea pigs and they were still dying. I didn't want to be a guinea pig. I didn't want to trust this doctor although I felt like he was really sincere in his actions. He was very supportive. He said, "You are HIV-positive. You have two and a half, three hundred something T-cells." He says, "You have under 500 T-cells. You need to get on AZT." I says, "Really, what about my tonsils?"

I really was against it but I took it anyway 'cause I thought, well, maybe I should do something. That's when I really started to feel that I was infected. My body was like tired all the time. I was nauseous. I was dizzy. So after two weeks I told them I was not taking it any more. I said I felt better without that. He says, "Well, OK it's your choice."

But I still wanted to go to the doctor often. I didn't want to take anything, but I still wanted to see the doctor once a week. So I got my tonsils out and my lymphs were swollen and I said to him, "What is this?" And he said, "Your body is probably infectious so they're going to be swollen." He says, "But you really need to worry when they go down. That means that you are close to the end." I said, "Well, how long is that going to take?" He said, "About a year." This was in March of '90. So from when he told me, I thought I had a year to live and I flipped out.

Cynora Jones Then, there was a wonderful doctor who prescribed me AZT. I was definitely allergic to it. You know, it just ached everywhere. My tongue swoll up where I was talking (*slurs words*) just like tttthhhiss. So he changed me to DDI. (*Laughs.*) I was running into walls, literally, and I'd watch my body spasm. And I said, This is not for me. (*Laughs.*) If this is a cure, I think I'll do without it.

Nancy Lemoins When I was really sick I stopped bleeding for a year. I know a lot of women have like pre-cancer stuff, yeah absolutely. I never had anything, you know. Also, the yeast that men get in their mouths, women get vaginally . . . Generally, I've had really good luck with doctors. I just found this really amazing woman a long time ago.

"We've got to stop guessing."

Marija Mrdjenovic Everyone is stuck in the past. It's the way that they've always done it, the way that they feel is the only way it should be done. And it's just as barbaric, it's just as tortured, it's as unnecessary as any of the so-called cures of the past. We shouldn't be looking for a drug answer; we shouldn't be looking for a vaccine answer. We should be looking at the human body and seeing how individual it is, how every individual has a different genetic makeup, how every individual has a different way of staying alive. We recognize distinctions in terms of ages with children and elderly people; their age is taken into consideration. But for some reason we still treat women as half-men, and expect them to have the same dosages as men, the same results as men, the same reactions as men. It's just not happening. If the doctors and if the researchers could finally just come together and say, "We were wrong. We were wrong; let's try this route, let's try helping the body help itself." A lot of the alternative therapists are saying that, but what they are offering is just herbal remedies. There's nothing wrong with a herbal remedy; it'll certainly not give you side effects like a drug will. But by the same token, it's a guess too. We've got to stop guessing about what's going wrong with the body. We've got cars. We put gas in the tank because we know that if we put sugar or something else in the tank it'll destroy the car. But we're willing to put sugar in the tank in people. We're willing to really screw up the whole immune system because we don't understand it. The immune system can provide answers that people have never dreamed of.

The profit motive

Raoul Thomas Oh there are so many conspiracy theories around AZT that not only I have thought of. Lots of people I know who are now since dead talked about the kickbacks the doctors would get for all the prescriptions they wrote, also kickbacks for information that they don't give as well as the prescriptions that they do write.

Nancy Lemoins I just have to tell you about this thing that happened last night. Along with the DeYoung [Art Museum], it was the biggest example of censorship I have experienced. I was at this panel and we were paid to talk about anti-viral medication, except that those of us who had said we were anti-drugs were totally shut out. We were not allowed to speak at all. I was paid to come there to speak but once they found out where I stood I wasn't able to make a point anywhere. They just let those who believed in them talk about them.

There is this drug they just came up with, it's a cure for like whatever makes you go blind. You use such small amounts of this drug and it's so cheap that they won't even put it on the market. That's insane. I really hate how this whole AIDS thing has become an industry and it's so far apart from what people need. It scares the shit out of me. It's like me and this protease inhibitor; I have such mixed feelings about being on this drug. I really, my legs hurt a lot. I'm really tired and that bothers me. I think they're really abusing us.

"No idea of the effect of the treatments."

Cynora Jones That was a month of taking anti-retrovirals and from that I now have peripheral neuropathy, damaged nerves on my right side because of medication, OK.

Philip Blazer It was Cinco de Mayo, May 5th, three years ago maybe. I was coming back from Civic Center. Septra and Vactrum are sulphuric drugs. I had had a reaction to them and I had to pull over. It hit me so fast and so hard to the point where I was losing control of the car. I just stopped my Volkswagen in the middle of the street and went over to Dolores Park and lay down in the park. I was there for about twenty or thirty minutes and someone who saw me came up and said, "They're going to tow your car." I lived nearby so I drove home. My roommate tended to me the rest of the day and evening. I had the chills, the sweats, the high fevers, aches, putting ice packs all over me. Finally I went to the emergency room. I was in a great deal of pain.

Marija Mrdjenovic But to get from here to there it's gonna take a lot more people screaming at them, basically saying "These drugs are not answers. We want to see something that will actually help our bodies." Antibiotics do not help the body. The combination therapies have killed so many people. I was taking at one point ten different drugs! But as long as I've stayed off of drugs, I feel better. The problem is here that doctors do not believe that you can survive AIDS if you go off the drugs. They will never ever see the harm that those drugs have done. Never.

And the drugs that they give you. With Septra, they give you the drug, see if you have a nasty side effect, and then take you off of it. Did you ever see the movie *Death Becomes Her*? She's given this potion so that she's going to be beautiful forever, but that she will need to be repaired over time. And they tell her the side effects after she's drunk it. And she goes, "Now you tell me? Now?" (*Laughs.*) And it's like that.

Just because a drug has a good effect doesn't mean that we should disregard a bad one. Treatment is something that does not give you side effects; it should be something that nourishes. Treatment is something that does *not* make you sick. (*Laughs.*) It's like the adage, "The operation was a success but the patient died." That's what's going on here.

Cynora Jones It's just more of man's inhumanity to man. You've got the Tuskegee Episode (Ji-Ahante Sibert, 1994). I liken it to this. I've had a lot of problems that could have been corrected. I was going to a male doctor and instead of him pushing for me to get the operation, he sedated me for two years on codeine Fours. Eventually I had to have a total hysterectomy. I'm looking at this – silence them, sedate them and maybe they'll go away. It's because of lack of education and because we look at doctors as gods.

Evolving doctor/patient relationships

Many lost faith in their doctors when the death prognoses did not materialize. Many of those PWAs lived years after diagnosis. In response, PWAs and AIDS advocacy organizations have challenged the conventional power dynamics of the doctor/patient relationships (Emke, 1993). The culture evolves and structures adapt. Currently the medical establishment is loosening up its orthodoxy; medical alternatives are gaining respectability (Brown, 1995; Verghese, 1995).

As the years of the disease continued with few medical breakthroughs, PWAs realized they needed to take more responsibility for their own treatments. Information became available for people with AIDS about how to best take a proactive role in their treatments (Project Inform, 1994). PWAs learned they could not blindly stop following the advice of doctors. Through the epidemic, doctors began listening more to the needs of patients. AIDS has brought an evolution of the doctor/patient relationship (Cohan, 1996; Mirken, 1995).

Robert Boulanget This was all in the time of Rock Hudson dying and being very sick and you saw it. You saw the face of AIDS on TV. On TV, you heard what everyone did in bed. That was the first time. Before that, maybe here in San Francisco they were a little bit more open to talking about the gay life, but nowhere else. That's one thing AIDS has done. Is it good or bad? It opens up everything. It opened the closet. It opened up sex. It opens up the way people treat their doctors and behave with their doctors. The doctor/patient relationship, it changes all that completely. You take charge of yourself. Doctors never had that before. It was always, you watch TV, all the programs they say, "You need to be in the hospital tomorrow. We're taking your tonsils out and that's it," and you do it. And now with AIDS people, a lot of them say, "No I don't want this; I'm not going to do that and I know what I want for myself." It definitely has changed that. It has changed the way people get better drugs because of ACT UP. And even other sicknesses are doing the same thing as AIDS activists. They're dealing with it the same way.

Mark Stanger Everyone said, if you come to San Francisco, the only place to get medical care is Ward 86 at General, whether you have insurance or not, go to General. So I did that, and that was one of the better experiences of my life. In very depressive, peely surroundings I met J. B. Molligan, the nurse practitioner, and I would feel pretty terrified. I would sit there and shake and sweat on the examining table. He would touch me and I would jump. In a few short medical visits he really helped my attitude. When he felt that I should start AZT, I didn't want to do that and I said, "Well maybe I will be on a study," but my blood work wasn't right for that and so he insisted that I start it and I said, "What if it makes me sick?" and I was really afraid. It was really funny. And then I said, "Do I have to back up the car to pick up all these pills?" 'cause I just couldn't imagine. And he said, "Well, if you cut the drama by about a half, we'll get it," and I needed to hear that. And the other thing, I kind of went into one of my frenzies and it's a kind of, in the stages of grief, it's a bargaining stage where I suddenly was going to adopt this perfect diet. I always had eaten pretty well but also enjoyed my Häagen-Das, so I was going to give up cappuccino. I start every morning with a latte, a very strong espresso left over from my early days. So I said I was going to give that up and he said, "Do you like that?" And I said, "I really like that." And he said, "Well then what do you expect to benefit? What is the benefit going to be by giving that up?" I thought, "Well, coffee's a toxin and it takes away vitamins and all this." And the last thing he said to me that meant so much, was at one point he said "It is OK to be freaked out from time to time. You don't have to like this every moment." It sounds just like psycho-babble, but he really gave me permission to have my feelings.

SEVENTEEN

Living Long-term with HIV

A large number of the migration cohort of San Franciscans underwent hepatitis testing in the late 1970s. Several interviewees participated in that study, years later had the blood tested, and found those samples to be HIV-positive. There are specific definitions of "Long-term survivor," according to the CDC. Living long-term with HIV has more to do with the simple idea of putting together quality years with HIV. Some researchers call those who have tested positive for HIV without progressing to AIDS, "nonprogressors" (Simmons, 1995). Theories abound as to how and why some live long-term with HIV. Some suggest it is genetic (Altman, 1996J; "Health," 1996); others that it is luck. Today's protease inhibitor cocktails allow those fortunate enough to have health insurance to stay alive. Those without are left to fend for themselves. Until protease inhibitors, which have yet to prove their effectiveness in the long term, few useful treatments existed.

Many were brazen enough not to take any medication when prodded by doctors. "Is it going to kill the HIV?" Darnell asked. "No." "Then why should I take it? When you have a cure, I'll take it. Until then, I'll take my chances." Others choose to take the drugs. A key tenet involves learning how the body functions, listening to that and responding. For some it involves finding a *raison d'être*: be it a great novel, activism, or faith. Again, health insurance doesn't hurt. Living long-term with HIV is one way of putting it, another would be just learning how to live. Interviewees reflect on their notions of living long-term with HIV.

Jay Segal There are tons of articles about the long-term survivors and what they have in common. They all have a belief system; they all have a support group; they all have religious, more like spiritual beliefs; they all have close families; they've got a good health care network; they're well educated, middle-class with lots of money.

Hank Wilson I've always gotten off seeing people be part of the resistance. To me the concept of resistance, even if we all end up dying, I think it's real important that there be a resistance that made its mark and that got its chips in, in terms of history.

Cleve's tips for long-term survival

Cleve Jones

> Avoid self-help books.
> Avoid the cure-of-the-month club.
> Avoid large amounts of alcohol or tobacco.
> Avoid nasty drugs.
> Eat well.
> Fall in love as often as possible.
> Have as much sex as possible.
> Enjoy life as much as possible.
> Keep your life decisions separate from your disease decisions (I didn't start taking any medicine at all until the last week of November).
> Don't let the disease rule you.
> Push your limits.
> Try consciously and actively, every day of your life, to do something to increase solidarity and to resist any isolating aspects of any disease.

That's what I've always tried to do.

I think it's very important to avoid cynicism and mysticism. These are really easy traps for people. So many people want to be cynical about the red ribbons. Just recently, I was coming home and one of the security personnel at the metal detectors had a red ribbon. I just said, "You know, I want to thank you for wearing that. I have AIDS and I appreciate knowing that you care about me." You can be cynical if you want. Sure, you know, life sucks; it's a cruel world, but I am so loved by so many people. To receive that kind of love and not acknowledge anything cheats the thing. I find ways every day of reminding myself that I am not alone, that there are a lot of really intelligent, compassionate people out there who really do care, and Newt is going to shoot himself in the foot any day now. Also, I am only forty and my God, what I have seen change, just for gay people, what I've seen change. It's incredible, absolutely incredible.

I got to preach in Rosa Parks' church. She made a quilt. One of the families on her block, three generations were killed by AIDS; the grandmother got it following a transfusion following hip surgery. Her daughter had been a drug user and a prostitute and had passed it on to the baby. Ms. Parks made a quilt for this family. I got to go to Detroit and to sit next to her and go out to lunch with her. That was like, if Dr.

King had come back or John Kennedy or somebody, well, that would be about as exciting. I had heard about Ms. Parks growing up and in Quaker meetings. Ms. Parks was given as an example of somebody who had followed the inner light and how one person, even if they are a small tiny person, can really change things. To meet her was very exciting.

Hank Wilson *Commenting from the Ambassador, a hotel housing PWAs, which he manages:* Some people will be long-term survivors like I am right now. I could be dead within I don't know. I would like to think that I'm going to make it through, but I also have a sense of humor about the whole thing. I believe in multiple lives. If you believe in multiple lives that's very convenient in the middle of this epidemic. I think that some of the people here will die and some of the people will survive. Some of the people here will be addicted. It's fascinating to work in a place and to have AIDS and to be around eighty people with AIDS. I've seen hundreds of people who have come through here and hundreds have already died. I've also seen people come in and they're already lining up on the floor and then they get inspired by me and by some of our other staff people who have AIDS. We don't give up. It's also a mind trip for some of them to find out, well he had AIDS and he's still working full time. Maybe I don't have to just throw my hands up.

Jay Segal If you lose your will to live you will die in three days. You've gotta stay positive. You've got everything within your power to do that. I've gotten cocky because I am on at least my seventh lifetime and I don't care. I don't know why, but I've gotta make it through this.

Entering your bliss

John Cailleau When the T-shirt fabric ended, that was the close of that chapter of the Castro where everything was wonderful. It was time for me to do something else. After moving into a cheaper place I got into the event business. Living with AIDS and the first few years of knowledge of this weird mysterious thing was relatively easy for me. The work I was doing was so incredible. I was finally doing for the first time in my life what I had always wanted to do, being a set designer in a public relations and marketing environment. The satisfaction of being an artist kept me going. It seems to me that the key to survival with this is to keep the internal energies, the creative force within us moving out, flowing, and flowering.

Just instead planting a seed and watering it and letting the suckers grow and doing it. I think the continued production and nurturance of that life energy is as important as AZT. It is a fucking test because the unpopularity of, number one, being gay and then later being gay and being HIV. Living with HIV has pushed me to begin moving from a physically oriented to a spiritually oriented life.

Spirituality plays a very big role in my coping mechanisms as well as my active creative mechanisms. When I realize that the power of intention and persistent will proves as a result – I have a very spacy metaphysical explanation for this stuff. If I'm connected to the universe with the spirit of creation and joy rather than with resentment and anger, the power of my intentions transfers over into that God. Since God then has the power to create the reality in the physical world, my intention communicated through that bridge of positive energy then creates changes within this great universal unconsciousness.

Positive attitude = life?

Nancy Lemoins It's hard to not go too far with the positive attitude = life thinking. When my friend David was dying, I mean David was really sick; he was blind. His ex-boyfriend showed up and said, "Oh David, it's your attitude. You don't have to die." I just was like, "My God, how fucking rude of you." His defense 'cause he was HIV too. He looked at David and said, "I don't have to be that way." It was fucked up. I think for people to go, it's just attitude or it's how much you try or it's how good you are is really wrong. I'm not saying that it's completely unimportant but you can't get too carried away. You can't blame yourself for being sick and go, "Oh I didn't try hard enough to be well" or go, "Oh, I wasn't spiritual enough" or nobody would ever die.

Jay Segal Everybody asks me how I get along this well. I'm T-42 negative. I do not have active virus in me. I have, obviously, a very slow and non-virulent strain of the disease. My T-cells went from 79 to 250 to 249. Fuck, I'm doing something right. I wish I knew. The standard line I use on the hotline is, "If I was in some state and it was a huge flowing river, really swift current, and there were thousands of people on the other side, I sure would like to know where the stepping stones are to get across."

Paul Greenbaum I'd probably be dead if I hadn't tried interferon six years ago. I may not quite have made it to being an interferon poster boy. My doctor said I'm one of his most successful patients. You have to be stubborn to want to persist with some of the frustrations.

The war and its impacts, its life lessons

Peter Groubert   *Groubert was stationed in Alaska when he was drafted in 1965 and nearly died in an explosion.* Going through a life-threatening situation definitely changed my life. I saw the world in a new perspective. Almost dying once, it was strange to have that happen, although I had no idea that it affected my life until many years later. HIV, it's another life-threatening thing. I was almost burned to death once in the army and now here I am again. I've been through it already. I'm not afraid of dying. If I were to die today, I'd just miss movies and TV. I'm up with all of my people. I think I've kissed and hugged everybody the last time I saw them, so . . .

Grace

Nancy Lemoins   My spirituality has changed a lot. You know, I've always been pretty spiritual but I lost my faith a lot when I was using. I think that was the only way that I could use was to let go of what was important. I tried really hard to die. I really was very lost, really dark. And today I am such a different person. I think going through that was absolutely not of my will, in fact, so totally against my will. I just don't hear. To come out of the other end of that and go it's not even up to me, hard as I tried. It just gave me my faith back. I think I kind of live in a state of grace. I don't take any credit for it on any level.

Arthur Fisher   Spirituality has been a sustaining thing most of my life. I had religious experiences when I was a kid and I learned very quickly that you don't talk about those things. It's gone from beliefs that help me, experiences that are valid, to more of what I do with my life. It was part of this last move. I was removed; actually I was thrown out of the hospice because I was too well. (*In a happy voice.*) They shared it with a Zen center where I turned out getting a room in the attic. I said to a friend, "This is really horrible; all I can do is pray and meditate. It's all you can do here." She turned around and said, "That's not so bad." Exactly. (*Laughs.*) I hadn't thought of that because I was too busy beating myself up and filling myself up with these judgments.

I can talk of chakras and I can talk of parallel existences, but they are all just worlds that I believe are made up to make us feel more secure. Well, we are not secure . . . If I can work up some massive intellectual idea that can make me understand that's nothing. I don't understand anything. When I'm comfortable in this position, it's the best place to me. It's also the most anxiety producing. I end up thinking I am crazy, I am out of my mind. But, I have been happily out of my mind often enough to know that that's OK, and my anxiety-ridden, out-of-my-mind phase passes. I've seen it enough times to be able to stand back or above or to the side and to be able to realize this is just my monkey under my ego going crazy and it'll go and I'll be fine.

A tanka on the wall

In China and Japan, there is Quan Yin, an entity, personage, Goddess, whatever you want to call it, who is compassion. One translation of the name is "she who hears the cries of the world." Quan Yin actually goes through, in history, a number of changes in gender and appears as a male, appears as a female. Quan Yin is hearing and giving out blessing . . . in a constant state of compassion, a constant hearing and response. I feel inspired and connected to that particular energy or thought. The face on the dresser across the room is Quan Yin from a temple in China that was destroyed during the Cultural Revolution. It was dug up in a field. There is something about that just as a state of being that is inspiring to me.

Beyond AIDS as cause and effect

I haven't resolved using illness as a teacher, using it as motivation, using crisis as motivation. It has been for me and for myself but I don't want to glamorize it, living through crisis, glowing through injury, wounded healer stuff. Yes, that happens. But I don't want to set it up as an ideal because then you have to get more wounded. If you want to be more enlightened, you have to be more wounded. If you want to be more loving, you have to be more hurt. I don't believe that I need that. Horror, pain and fear are blessings and will help you grow. No, that's not it! It's getting out of it that helps, not it. There is no glamour in pain and fear and trauma and disease.

I don't know how much of my early trepidations were societal programming that just constantly, just relentlessly pounds in that this is the way life is, that this is the way the world is. My last experience in the hospice when I came back from Mexico, the KS was bad and I couldn't walk without a great deal of pain in my legs. My feet were swollen and painful. Actually I had KS in my throat and my face. I didn't go out. I hemorrhaged in my throat and realized maybe I could hemorrhage in a major organ so this could be it. I was in and out of consciousness and had this experience with what seemed to be my future self at the time.

Second dance. I knew somehow that there were things that I had to do and I set to doing them and I got better. I was really proud of that, and ended up going through a program for self-empowered people with HIV and tried to help other people to do it . . .

This last time that I got very sick, I got meningitis. I don't remember a good deal of it. Very painful. I moved back into the hospice. I came out of the hospital and came home, couldn't take care of myself, collapsed again, went back to the hospital and was told that I needed twenty-four-hour care. So I understood that this time I wasn't to wish myself alive or to wish myself dead, and, being a control freak at heart, that was a frustrating thing. Now I want to make a decision, "OK, OK, everyone, I am going to die now. I'm in control and this is my decision." But this was not about doing that just be here, meditate and pray and forgive and be here and that's all. And I got better. I knew that with this matter, I didn't have anything to do with it. I did in the respect that I got out of my own way and I listened. I let go of things, but I didn't do it any more than medicine heals or cures anybody. I can remove things to let the body heal itself, that let help and balance come. A lot of that fog went away. A lot of it's still here but a lot of it went. It's not control. It's not being able to overcome, it's also not being a victim. It's not all of those roles.

Ronnie Ashley I think I've made it this far, not just with HIV, but all my life, through humor and having a positive attitude about everything I do. I acknowledge the stupidness, the ignorance, the hatred, the ugliness. But then I turn around and find out what was positive, take that with me and move on. And I'm not dying with HIV, I am living with HIV. I ain't ready to go there. And I don't like people telling me, "No, you can't do that; you gotta take this." Uh-uh, each individual has to be true to themselves. You gotta know where you're coming from, where you're going, where you're headed, doing what you came from, Sister, all the way around. I think that it's very important that you seek a balance mentally, physically, spiritually and emotionally. Because it's who you are and what you are and a big part of how you exist in that cycle. We continue to eat all these foods; these are just souls that continue to recycle themselves into our existence and who we are as human beings and spirits walking on this earth. We all got our horror stories and our atrocities. We all have our histories of ugliness, racism, genocide, but it cannot end there. We still have work to do.

There's a saying among my people that your riches are not necessarily measured by what you have as much as by what you give away.

Volunteerism teaches you about giving away. But the things that you receive are unmeasurable.

Never in my wildest dreams would I ever think that someday, here I am, I am going to retire some time, only because of my HIV. I always used to think, God, man I hope I live as long as my grandmother. I gotta live as long as my grandmother. My grandmother died when she was 103. I always wished. I remember when I was younger, I always hoped I'd live as long as she did because here was a woman that was born in 1880 and was just brought up in a whole different world than what I know now, no cars and electricity and stuff and seeing all that evolution and that that ran by her. I always felt, God, I hope I live to be 103 and have my own history. And even as I look back, being forty-three, I have a lot of history. I've been through a lot of history and I continue to rebuild history, continue to make a contribution and I have to acknowledge, "yes, you made a contribution." In this ugly climate that is AIDS work you often don't hear that, even though you feel that other part of the world and those gifts that you receive from your clients and from your volunteers and from the people that you work with and those that die and move on.

David Pattent   I literally have this visualization process that I use to communicate with my virus. I gave my virus a physical being. And I have this dialogue with my virus, essentially. And notice I say my virus. I own that. It's not *the* virus, or *a* virus, it is *my* virus because it is in my body. Essentially, the dialogue goes, "Virus, you're powerful, you can kill me. Virus, I'm powerful. I can kill you. All I have to do is take some pills, and you're history. Now what's the purpose of that? We both have one instinct: survival. And we will do whatever it takes to survive. So if you kill me off you're essentially killing yourself off. If I kill you, I'm killing me. So why don't we just sort of coexist?" And we can coexist. We have very effectively coexisted together. "Two conditions: Don't try and kill me, because if you try and kill me I will kill you. I *will* win. I don't want to do this win/lose thing. Let's not do that, let's just both be okay with where we're at. And the second condition is that you're not going to leave my body. I'm not going to give you to somebody else, I'm not going to allow you to procreate."

I've switched a whole way of thinking around to "Today is the last day of my life. Am I complete with everyone? Have I done all the things that I wanted to do with my life, based on what I've got to work with right now?" Yes I have. So if I drop dead tonight, I could be very content. I wouldn't want anyone saying "Oh that poor person, he died so young and didn't lead a full life." I've had an amazing fucking life. I can't resent that. And I want more. And if I don't have it, I'm OK with that. If I woke up tomorrow morning and found out that I have twenty-four hours to live, I would be OK with that. It's not about, "Oh my God there are so many things I still want to do." And I won't feel that I've been deprived; I don't feel that I've ever been robbed of anything. I don't feel that HIV has done anything but have a positive impact on my life. And that's the way I viewed it literally since day one.

PART VI

Fragmentation

EIGHTEEN

Left vs. Left: The Clinton Years

With the election of Bill Clinton, the Concord Data acknowledging AZT's limited usefulness, and a new wave of infections (Gross, 1993; Rofes, 1996: 3), the AIDS pandemic entered a second generation with few more answers than were available during the previous decade. Certain assumptions by doctors and activists characterized the first decade. Assumption number one that a "magic bullet," the discovery of a cure, was in reach in the near future failed. Activists built tactics around assumption number one. They fought for accelerated approval and affordable access to new drugs, such as AZT. Many of these, however, proved counterproductive. Assumption number two suggested that from 1981 to 1993, Reagan and Bush were the demons of the AIDS epidemic. Their neglect motivated activists. Though Clinton's response was ineffective and far more enigmatic, AIDS was not born under his watch.

As the epidemic evolved and became more complex, focus among AIDS groups was lost in part because of the loss of common enemies, death-based attrition, and the ever elusive nature of the virus (Kolata, 1995). From 1992 to 1995 AIDS activism became exhausted and in need of reassessment. Fissures reflecting the larger society showed (Radosh, 1996). Debilitating infighting among the left and its counterproductive effect on the AIDS movement is the subject of this chapter.

AIDS and the culture of division

On more than one occasion, Freud explained that he could deal with his enemies, it was his friends who worried him (Gay, 1988: xvii). In the age of Clinton and America's diverse society, Freud's sentiment cannot be underestimated. The first two years of the Clinton Administration were a battle against division (Lind, 1996). The left vs. the left, a national phenomenon, plays a major role in the history of the San Francisco AIDS epidemic. From the Bathhouse Closure to the Shanti Scandal, to rejection of Clinton over Gays in the Military, infighting has played a debilitating spoiler role. Liberals snipe at the ankles of other liberals. They battle over the leftovers of the gutted budgets while right-wingers rub their hands with satisfaction. By 1994, with the loss of the Democrat-controlled Congress, internal struggles and missed opportunities in San Francisco act as a microcosm of the failure of the national Democratic left.

Infighting among the left has deep roots in San Francisco (witness Tom Wolfe's *Mau-Mauing the Flak-Catchers* (1970), chronicling dynamics between Bay Area "community organizers" and "poverty bureaucrats" a generation ago). Today, the ethnically diverse coalition battling on the many fronts of the AIDS war teeters. When everyone in a coalition has his or her own individual self-concepts and group histories, it is difficult to fight for common goals (Cafferty and Chestant, 1976). AIDS activists have grown resistant to adapt away from their assumed roles. Gitlin (1995) explains, we are living in an era of "the twilight of common dreams." The division of the AIDS movement reflects a larger trend. Firestone (1976) writes that during the 1960s, America evolved into a diverse society of interests bringing about a death of common cause:

> Their view of their society as a cohesive organic whole, dedicated to the pursuit of common goals was increasingly replaced by an image of America as a mosaic of diverse groups, each with its own separate goals and its own insistent demands for justice, equality and freedom. The belief that public life was based upon consensus was belied by the emergence of many competing perspectives. The issues of the Cold War increasingly shared the political stage with issues generated by the internal divisions of American society.

Internal divisions, friends, and demons

These internal divisions created the politics of AIDS and made management of the AIDS agenda in the era of ongoing epidemic extraordinarily difficult. These divisions (and poor management) (Kreiger, 1996) helped bring about the near death of Shanti Project, one of San Francisco's oldest AIDS service agencies, which took the brunt of a decade's accumulation of frustration. At the same time, the real enemies – disease, homophobia, lack of a cure, inadequate health care, a void of national leadership, and evolving demographics – roared unchecked. Shanti Project was a friend; the scandal surrounding it represented a depressing culmination of the first generation of a response to the epidemic. Infighting around policies, ranging from bathhouse closures, prevention messages, or ACT UP zapping sympathetic audiences, represents a long shadow of the AIDS story (Odets, 1995; Associated

Press, 1989; Carrol, 1991). Failure to distinguish between friends and enemies bubbled to a high pitch as the Clinton years continued without a cure in sight (Ford, 1995; Tuller, 1993). The community had lost sight of priority number one: ending the epidemic (Jones, 1995).

Priority number one

Jay Segal I have the utmost respect for it. It's a virus and that's all it is. There's only one enemy. It's not the government or George Bush or Ronald Reagan or any of them, it's the virus, that's it. You've gotta remain focused that there is only one enemy.

Reagan and his critics

Arthur Fisher I think Republican cooperation as the epidemic began was along the lines of annihilation. I think we went through years of neglect. There's a certain amount of it now but, I mean, it was intense. This last presidential election was the first time I ever voted. It got too scary to think we could end up with Bush for another four years. That was massive hatred going on. There is this consolidation of Republicans and the Christian Right. It was dangerous, dangerous for poor people.

In terms of fighting that, it's a hard one for me to try to determine when some part of my ego wants to say when to lower to someone else's level. When do you have to do that? I don't know. I wish that we had a number of very strong, intelligent and compassionate leaders in the community with Gandhian appeal and clarity instead of blind rage. Perhaps blind rage is better than blind submission, but I'd rather address the blindness than the rage or the submission. You know, to not let the society trample us, and to try to engage in a different way rather than lowering to blind rage. Sometimes that's not possible and I don't know what to do with that . . . You could drown waiting for clarity.

Blind rage, ACT UP, and enduring legacies

John Cailleau I think that they have done an effective job on getting those drugs out into the marketplace that normally wouldn't have been out there because they were "too dangerous." I mean, if you are going to die of something anyway. But I disagree with instances where they went to the opera house and unveiled a banner and just raised holy hell there. I don't think they have done a good job distinguishing between friends and enemies. They would go to a friendly environment and create some disruption to get the attention and probably piss more people off because of the tactic rather than the message.

Raoul Thomas Even towards the beginning, there was more hope for a cure. Now the most you hear about is talk for a vaccine. I think first the population who is not infected will probably receive some sort of a vaccine maybe by the year 2000, 2010. By then it's already too late; it'll be definitely too late for me. That sums up my politics as well.

There's so much anger around that, I don't know, you can't kill people, but who, who is to blame? Who is responsible? There is no answer there. The rage is there. But anger has a way of turning itself into so many other destructive forces, but more so self-destructive. It turns itself inward with fear and outward with hopelessness. It feeds on itself too and once you start getting angry, you can get angry about a lot of stuff. But anyone who does anything towards the battle against AIDS deserves a medal because it's a real war. The things that make me angry about it are the little stop-gap things like the ribbons and the red ribbon stamp. Will that save me?

Hazel Betsey The attack always goes in the wrong place. You attack your own for some reason. It's like in the riots, blacks attacked the blacks. They burnt down their own neighborhoods in a riot that was supposed to have been against the white man who was against us. And we ended up hurting ourselves. All cultures seem to do that. They attack the lesser ones. You start fighting yourselves and so you get nowhere.

"SILENCE = DEATH" as a twentieth-century icon – the attrition point

G'dali Braverman I think that within the history of all political movements there are divisions and subdivisions. I think that movements become fortified and watered down as they grow. You can look at the history of political theory and what happens. History really does repeat itself. You see it over and over again, whether it's the Black Panthers or whether it's SDS or whether it's ACT UP. People do not come into a movement that are essentially of like minds. People come into a movement because they have, essentially, the same interest in the same issue. But their origins are completely different. The key is how to, how do you use that diversity without letting it dissect the organization. I think there are inevitabilities of splits and I think that they need to happen and they can be healthy. But I think also sometimes splits happen and conflicts within an organization are almost like a disease itself; it's almost that the body is fighting all these cancer cells and it's going through its own triage and the body begins fighting itself. That's what happens within organizations. Friends turn into enemies and people turn against each other and divisions become blurred.

I, me, mine and a culture of division and atrophy

Peter Groubert   There were so many great, great people, truly powerful people, people that really cared. People like Bill Kraus and many others of that vein. There are no leaders now. There's no one charismatic person who can gather the community. Forget about that you are black or you are yellow, you're a man or a woman; we're gay and we have something we need to do. Follow me and I'll get us through this. There is nobody like that now. People won't follow. You know, Harvey was one of those people. Kind of sad, the only legislation he ever got passed in his short time, The Pooper-Scooper Law.

Hazel Betsey   One thing that bugs me with this city is the groups. Sometimes I feel like I should go to African-American HIV support groups or African-American recovery groups. But I am not a separatist. When I have gone to HIV-positive groups that are all men, I feel a part of those men because we are infected. They didn't make me feel unwelcome but I knew that I also needed to get support from women. I wish that there wasn't so much "this group," "that group" type stuff going on. Even in the gay world, certain gay people like to stay with their own.

Robin Tichane   AIDS has been such a big issue, I won't say that the various things that little groups are doing, that that energy is not doing fabulous things, they really are, but it's decentralized, and that's the way politics wants it in this city. They want things to go that way because it means more power for them rather than more power for an organized, coherent gay community. It has lost a lot of the focus.

Raoul Thomas   I'd like to say there was something really positive about being positive, that it was somehow bringing people together or unifying families. But I don't know. You hear more stories about division. It can put an enormous wedge between people. It has happened to me. I've seen more wedges than I have togethernesses.

Wedges within the community: bathhouse closures

Hank Wilson and Cleve Jones, both long-time gay activists, comment on the days in the mid-'80s when, for health reasons, a number of Liberationists advocated closing down the San Francisco bathhouses (Shilts, 1987: 339–495). They both recall the McCarthy Era tactics used against them by activists with differing views.

Hank Wilson On the bathhouse thing, I have the distinction of being on the Enemies List in *Bay Area Reporter*. I was one of the fifteen people on the list. The list was put together against people that were supporting the bathhouse closure. Other people weren't talking to me either, which was another mind-fucker. You might have thought we were all in league, but that wasn't the case. I was frozen out. I worked to keep the bathhouses open in two different meetings with Merv Silverman, the director of public health, and then I changed. Previously I had argued that we could use the bathhouses as vehicles to educate people. The reality was the bathhouse owners were assholes. They would not allow us to put up signs, condoms, or anything. So when that became clear, I changed my mind. I said, "Fuck you; all you want is money." In the meantime, I was a heavy bathhouse goer. I was going all the time, which some of the other people weren't. And you could see what was happening in the bathhouses and people were not dealing with the context of the epidemic.

Cleve Jones The traitor list . . . and from the beginning there's just been horrendous, horrible division. We've seen more examples of it in the last few months: the split between the treatment activists on the whole issue of accelerated approval, the fight over unionization at the San Francisco AIDS Foundation, and this disruption of the Project Inform Dinner (see Swissler and Salinas, 1995; Rottcamp, 1995). It still goes on. I think that part of that is due to the fact that the gay community is such a bitchy community. Some people don't like it when I say that.

But when I was running for office, I went out and I collected copies of all of the ethnic and neighborhood newspapers in San Francisco. We've got French-language newspapers and Russian and Spanish and Filipino and Chinese and Japanese and Korean and every neighborhood has a newspaper. And I went through them all and only in the gay press did you find consistently, in issue after issue, in the letters to the editor section, vicious personal trashing by name of individual activists. You don't see it like you do in our community anywhere else. Expect internal fights.

Look at the NAACP, which has just been through an incredible leadership struggle, but not this kind of public trashing, crucifixion of leadership.

When Bill Kraus and Ron Huberman and I published the letter, Bill wrote it actually but I think Ron and I each edited it, but we wanted to write it as three single gay men who were sexually active who were part of the scene. We wanted people to know we weren't home in some cosy monogamous relationship. We were out looking too. We published this thing just suggesting that maybe we ought to cool it. People spat on me. They called me a Nazi fascist for even suggesting. People are incredibly nasty. It's weird for me. I have been subjected to so much abuse from these people. And you know what, in my whole life, I have been attacked once by straight people. I was attacked once by fag bashers in Sacramento and stabbed and nearly killed. But I've never had a letter to the editor from a straight person saying, "Oh, that Cleve Jones, he's a bad faggot. We don't like him." The letters I got have all come from gay people. I have been accused of all sorts of outrageous things and it's rough. They did it to Harvey too, especially the PC crowd, the ultra-leftists. I once had a party and people walked out of the party because Harvey was there. I'm getting hate mail right now because I am grand marshal of the Gay Rodeo. I'm getting hate letters from animal rights activists . . . It's very frustrating.

Stresses and the politics of AIDS

I went to Richard Chavez, then the Shanti activities director, for help in terms of finding interviewees. As we talked about putting an ad in the next Shanti Bulletin he mentioned that he would be interested in being interviewed, as he was positive.

We met at the Mobi Tobi Revolution Café in Hayes Valley. Richard, a confident man with a gray beard, long brown hair, and a customarily casual demeanor, wore a black T-shirt tucked into his jeans with a leather belt and belt buckle. At points his brown eyes strayed out the window; at others, he sat up with his hand on his chin. We smoked a lot of cigarettes, drank even more coffee and took on the contentious topic of the rise and fall of the Shanti Project. Once on the forefront of the internationally recognized service paradigm, the "San Francisco Model," Shanti Project fell into a streak of bad luck as combinations of innuendo, carnivorous political moods and dyslexic accounting made casual appropriations of funds take on the nuances of embezzlement. When the image of a Porsche and glamour lifestyle paid for with the scant portion of the ever-dwindling resource pie actually allotted to the pestilence-

besieged city came to the surface, whether true or not, a sore spot had been irritated. This was a community already reeling as they transitioned from the novelty of the Eros and Emancipation of the '70s to the painful, chronic multiple loss syndrome laden '90s. The press and community went on a feeding frenzy. Faith among funders and clients dissipated. Shanti was forced to forfeit programs. "It really stressed me out for one. I didn't know if I would have a place to live anymore," Nancy Lemoins, who was living at the Shanti House, recalled. Many mark the Shanti scandal as the nail in the already strained coffin of the "San Francisco Model" (Botkin, 1995). The backlash against Shanti is another example of the community failing to distinguish between friends and enemies. Richard reflected on the underlying politics of AIDS which brought about the scandal. (For background on the scandal see Sabin, 1992, 1993A, B; Tuller, 1993; Bay Area Report, 1993A, B; Moore, 1993A, B; Provenzano, 1993; Rojas, 1994; Pae, 1994; Garfield, 1995; Lee, 1996; Rofes, 1996: 34, 52–66).

Richard Chavez Discrimination comes from people making rules. Some organizations, for example, that provide services have decided that if you don't have a phone number, they can't help you. AIDS discrimination happens because of an economy. There's a level of economic discrimination going on. If you're not from a certain economic group or a value system, you can't be involved with certain groups. On the other side, the other political issue is if you're not from this ethnic group we can't help you; we'll send you to another agency and they can help you, ethnic interest. And that's another form of political stupidity. A lot of people on the board of directors at certain organizations are definitely people from a different economic class because they're able to bring in money and organize; that takes free time. Privileged people have free time to be on the boards and to dictate what their organization is going to be about and who is and is not going to be hired.

There were a lot of political favors being done in hiring until San Francisco got shook up by a lot of organizations having been caught on the griddle and told something's wrong. In the long run, there was just community consciousness that caused all these organizations to move from the grass roots to a little bit more organized, a little bit more accountability as to what they were doing and who they were. Economic prejudices were forced out. A lot of the serviced people came from the Tenderloin and that's good. You'd see the old groups, a lot of the old troops who were involved with AIDS organizations at the very beginning getting angry and writing letters about organizations because they have lost ground and they can't dictate what is going on in the AIDS community and who are getting services. It's the focus of their anger and frustration about themselves and what they're going through. They lash out on the most obvious thing, the organization that's helping, transference as they call it in psychology.

Wedges within the community: the Shanti scandal

Ronnie Ashley *The story of Shanti Project demonstrates the unfortunate consequences of a community's inability to distinguish friends from enemies.* I don't want to talk about the politics of Shanti Project. It sucks, sucks, sucks. What has happened to the agency over the years because of politics, because of money, because of people's own political agenda. It is the politics of AIDS and the money of AIDS that dictate what people will do. You have to play the political in order to get the money to serve the people. And all the agencies, in their heart and soul, came into it with this idea of giving something back to the community. We all started off as grass roots organizations but now it is big business.

Richard Chavez What happened was that we had some directors who were very much into providing services to people. Sometimes we needed money to do a training, for example for volunteers or something, and they would just take from the main source and pay for all the training and the food and the time and the salaries and blah, blah, blah. Whereas they were supposed to, should have written documentation on those things and put it into the AIDS Office, and the AIDS Office now says they would have approved that. Because that paperwork wasn't done. It wasn't the fault of Shanti. It was the fault of the accountants that we hired. When they would go through the books they would just say we need specifics on this and this, and then they would send it into the AIDS Office. I wonder myself and have my suspicions about who these people were and what connections they had . . . I don't know.

We paid the money back to the AIDS Office. The AIDS Office said, "All these things that you said you used for the housing programs would have been fine if you would have documented it and had us approve it." Our accountants needed to be on top of that, but they weren't. So we're working on this. I'm not sure about the outcome. I'm not privy to that information. That's what I have been told.

And someone had to pay for it. They blamed directors, the executive and the deputy executive director, and they had to give up their positions. Somebody had to pay for it because the community wanted blood and the board of directors wanted blood. The board didn't want to accept the responsibility, but they accepted it and moved on from there. People left the board and all the changes happened that needed to happen. They're all good people with the best of intentions, but then again the road to hell is paved with good intentions, isn't it?

There was no embezzlement because the AIDS Office came back with a press release in January this year saying, "Nothing really was wrong." Then people said, "Well why did everybody have to go through this? Why did good people have to leave Shanti? Why did we have to give up programs?" It's interesting, when this all hit the fan a lot of the other organizations who were on the AIDS Office Commission, some of the loudest critics saying, "You gotta take programs away from Shanti and close it down." Those programs were the ones that got these programs taken away. And guess what – it's a pain in the ass for them.

In the beginning, Shanti was forced to take the housing program and everybody else got scared. Shanti was becoming one of the biggest, budgetwise, groups. It went from a two million budget to five point something million a year as an organization, that's big. Some people got scared and saw the first sign of something wrong and everybody went, "Ahhh! We want the money back!" Well they got the money and now they're saying, "Hey, we can't do it on this money." "No kidding."

When people come in and say, "I was on the housing program at Shanti. I want to know what my status is," it's really sad to say, "We don't provide that service anymore and you need to talk to . . . ," and we give them the list of names. "You call this office first and let them know that you're concerned about your housing and then you call this group and then you call this program and then you call this foundation. These are the four that have the programs and they are the ones that you need to call." And the horror stories that I am hearing from clients about the new housing programs. The poorest part is that PWAs are fighting for their lives and they are the ones who have to suffer from all this garbage. They're the ones that come up short and they don't need this. It's really sad, that's draining, that's real draining, sort of sad.

Darnell Davis and Hugo Manzo, who both have lived in one of the Shanti buildings, comment in the chapter on AIDS Inc. Chavez went on:

The sad part of the AIDS story

Me, I guess it was inevitable if it was going on for so long . . . That's part of the sad thing about the AIDS story. When those organizations were formed, the KS Foundation, the AIDS Foundation, Shanti didn't think they were going to be coming into a lifetime AIDS organization. They were a cancer organization. Then there were all the activist problems and then you've got this Whitewater press feeding frenzy. Then the organization was doubling in money. GMHC is now two big buildings. It's a business thing and you have to be accountable to that.

I think the big lesson is that hidden agendas are no longer permitted, because they were permitted before. They were all under this guise of helping people. Now we have to be focused in on the clients as opposed to, "Well, we're going to get this thing going because we're all dying." No, we're living longer and you have to provide for the living situation now. We cannot permit the hidden agenda anymore. A lot of the board of directors, executive directors, whatever it is, big salaries; that's gone. It won't continue. That's what this is all about.

Ethnocentrism and hidden agendas

People were ready to move on to becoming less to do with being an AIDS advocate within AIDS organizations. The gay community can let them become the board of directors or supervisors in government, congressmen. There is something more. This is a stepping-stone for them. The ambition of being something rather than what they were doing, those are the hidden agendas.

Some of them are those that say, "Oh, you don't understand us because we're, whatever, we're Catholics. Our needs are different. We're going to start our own little organization . . ." People needed jobs and their hidden agendas came in there. They wanted to make a name for themselves too. Those are the same ambitions of being rather than doing. Those organizations don't exist anymore. Because the disguise of ethnicity was, "We're different so we have to do our own thing." Those are over with. That's a lie . . . hypocrisy.

My anger, I take it out at the gym. I get angry at boards of directors and those kinds of people. I get angry at Clinton. I think he's a liar. I get angry about the rules of AIDS organizations when I hear stories from people, my own experiences now from all organizations. Insurance companies I think are abominations. There are some real sins in the world and I think that we're committing those sins on people, cutting people's money income, which is from SSI or from disability? Come on. People are starving and they have AIDS. They don't have money to eat. They'd rather take the medication. I think that's where the anger comes from. I'm real angry about that.

A few of the real enemies

Ronnie Ashley Here we have a health care system that is totally crippled. It can't take care of the mass needs of the community. I'll use an example. The active substance-use community. You have to address their substance use before you can even get them services. In order to do that you've got to get them into detox. They've probably been homeless so you have to get them emergency shelter, hook them up into Medicare, Medicaid and so on and so forth. I can't get people into detox 'cause I got fucking detoxes that are on three- to six-month waiting lists. I can't get them housing 'cause I've got housing that is a three-year waiting list. I can get them a little bit of Medicare, but I just don't understand. I feel it is my human right to get all the medical attention that is out there.

G'dali Braverman The voices that I trust are what David Feinberg writes or what Larry Kramer writes, as much as some of it is not based in scientific reality, it's based in the truth of a rage. Most everyone else has fallen into some sort of bureaucracy that supports an AIDS industry.

NINETEEN

Health Care and the Death of AIDS Activism?

"We spend hours debating the merits of whether national health insurance should be one of our basic demands on every flyer we send out," David Feinberg (1994) wrote about his early years with ACT UP New York. Years later, a Democratic President proposed that very thing. Without a cure in sight, national health care had become the most pressing need for PWAs. The issue, however, had lost priority.

In his essay, "What Ever Happened to AIDS," Jeffrey Schmaltz (1993: 60) felt that the 1993 Gay March on Washington's concentration on the Gays in the Military issue reflected a drift; "AIDS was an element of the march, but just an element. Speaker after speaker ignored it." Few addressed the obvious need for health care for PWAs. In "United We Stand; Divided We Grovel: Queers and the Health Care Debate," McLarty (1994) argued that AIDS groups had lost sight of a common goal by putting so much effort into an issue like Gays in the Military which lacked unanimous support even among gays. Larry Kramer (1993A) argued: "I'm perplexed that it has become number one on the agenda of things for us to deal with when AIDS is so much more important . . . Why anybody gay or straight would want to serve in the armed forces is beyond me." Neither health care nor the military policy was reformed. And as an unintended consequence, these fights cost Democrats vital political capital nationally (Berke, 1996). Urvashi Vaid observed, "What we needed to learn from the military fight is that we have to build more political power before we win any gay issue on a national level" (Dunlap, 1996A).

No President had proposed such a comprehensive piece of social legislation since the Johnson Great Society years. Today, the possibility of comprehensive national health care feels like a dream. In July 1994, the twilight of the health care debate years, Mike Fandel, a long-term survivor of thirteen years, reflected on what he sensed was becoming a lost opportunity. We drank coffee outside in the sunny wood patio of Sweet Endings, a café on Church Street off Market. With an easygoing

Midwestern demeanor, Mike, a fit man with thinning sandy brown short hair parted down the middle, brown eyes behind wire-rimmed glasses, wearing a white Oxford shirt, suggested that a die may have been cast when his community failed to step to the plate in the national health care debate. Three months later Democrats lost control in Congress, having conceded defeat in the health care debate in early August. As the Roosevelt coalition was crumbling, only months before his own death, Mike articulated a view that would come to be a consensus (Skocpol, 1996; Daniels, 1995). He pointed out the central role national health care, the incomplete cornerstone of the New Deal, could play in the battle to make HIV a chronic manageable disease. With today's exorbitant costs (Altman, 1996C), Fandel's insight addresses the pressing AIDS issue.

G'dali Braverman was a member of David Feinberg's ACT UP old New York chapter, which argued for the central role of health care for PWAs, most of whom are gone now. By 1994, he looked like an anachronism when, wearing a T-shirt proclaiming "Have a Happy AIDS," he was arrested for taking over Senator Feinstein's office in protest at her failure to support the Mitchell Health Care Plan (Conkin, 1994). National health care was the battle most everyone chose not to fight.

Mike Fandel   Back in the era of Reagan and Bush, we had a clear enemy. We could become politically active and angry at these right-wing conservatives who, in our view, as gay men and PWAs, these were the enemy. We could become very reactionary and angry at them. Now things have been kind of diluted because when Clinton came into the White House, PWAs thought there was going to be a change and thought that here was somebody who was willing to do the right thing.

What surprises me is the lack of involvement on the part of AIDS activists on the health care issue. If there's one thing that has a direct impact on people with AIDS in the AIDS community, it is the Health Care Bill. Why are the leaders on AIDS activism not speaking out and becoming very active in support of Clinton and the Health Care Bill? It's like, why not? This is something that is going to have such a direct immediate impact on everybody with AIDS, and if you look at the costs.

Probably the reason why I'm sitting here is because I've had privileged health care. I had a company that I worked for that provided me with extremely good health coverage. I have access to the best doctors in San Francisco, the best that medical science can provide. But if I lose that health care coverage, which is a very real possibility since I'm no longer working, when that runs out, what then? Whose gonna pay for the $50,000 a year for one drug that I need? And I know that if I don't have this drug, I will be in the hospital; I will be sick; I will probably die without this drug. But it's $50,000 a year.

Of course, there's also that other issue: why is it costing so fucking much? (*Laughs.*) That's outrageous, that's prohibitive to many people. Why are the drug companies raping us for the cost of these drugs? It doesn't cost that much to make. What they're saying is that it costs that much to do the research to develop and they're trying to recoup their prior costs in developing it. When I first started taking AZT, it cost something like $25,000 a year. Now it's down to about $7,000.

Everybody with AIDS is going to have to deal with the health care system. (*Laughs.*) You have no choice. But I've heard nothing. I read the gay rags, the *BAR*, *The Sentinel*, and you see nothing about the community becoming involved. Why? The rallying cry is in access to health care. True, there is no one single AZT or one single magic bullet, but the rallying cry should be access to the full gamut to all people in similar situations as myself. Good quality health care in this country is a right, not a privilege. As it stands now it's a privilege. I'm part of the privileged class because I have good health care insurance.

It's almost like going through different stages. In the early years of the AIDS epidemic, we were going through the angry stage. We were pissed off that this was happening to us. We had to focus on the enemy; the enemy was Reagan, then Bush; the enemy was Boris Welcome and AZT. Now, it's much more complex. There are no simple enemies. What do we have to do? We've got to get over that angry stage and I think somewhat we are. That true activism anger has kind of died down and now we have to focus on the needs of people with AIDS, and that is good quality health care, helping people to make the right decisions for themselves, not getting on a bandwagon of the right thing for everyone to do 'cause there is no such thing. It's gonna be different for everyone, whether they are different for a black woman and a white man and even different for two white men. There is no one way to go with this. What needs to be done in my view is some sort of a foundation of good quality care, that and education that can allow people to make the right decisions for themselves. That's I think the most important thing. The anger and the hate, that's not going to work. It's understandable in the early years because we were all going, "My God, what's happening? Who's at fault? Who's to blame for this? Why isn't anybody doing anything about it?" And that's real understandable, but that's changing.

Where are the leaders in the AIDS community or I mean the gay community? Most of those people died. We don't have true leaders in the community, people that the whole community can rally behind.

Part of the reason is that even within the community there's so much conflict. You know, you've got the lesbians; you've got the blacks; you've got white males. And there's kind of pitting each group up against the other. Even if each of those groups might have leaders within them, none of those leaders can rise to be a leader over the whole community, so you get a diffusion of energy and power. In order to be focused politically, you have to be focused. Part of the problem with the gay and the AIDS community right now is there's no focus.

United we stand, divided we drift

Hank Wilson I want to be around. I want to fight it. I think when I look at my ACT UP group, we've got these cycles too in our group. Sometimes you need to ride it through, but sometimes it's important for people to keep together. I think sometimes we spend too much time fighting with people we disagree with and never coalesce with people. I remember when Vice-President Mondale came out here and we picketed him. The Democratic Party leadership, they were furious at us. We were supposed to be lucky that a sitting vice-president would come to our city and here we disrupted his cocktail party and we screamed. We did all these things. I remember them lecturing us but we waved our signs and blocked the shit out of him and our community divided. We are so lucky, I love history, I love to read history, to be at the right place but sometimes we like to coast a little and I feel like sometimes we do coast a little.

Postscript – the death of AIDS activism?

Cleve Jones What I thought last night walking in the Candlelight Memorial [the twelfth annual AIDS Candlelight Vigil] was so much about my friends who are gone. You know, it's kind of hard to describe what it's like to lose everybody you know, but that's what happened. The people who joined the struggle in ACT UP, many died, many of them got burned out, or have chosen to stay home to take care of themselves or others. Others have gotten jobs in the industry. As for what's happening now, what we are seeing is the accumulated toll of fifteen years of death. People like to talk about what's happened with ACT UP, but the single most fundamental thing with ACT UP is that they have died.

G'dali Braverman I think that AIDS activism as we know it is dangerously close to being on its deathbed. And I am not certain that it won't die as we know it. My prediction actually is that it will die as we know it and that several years will pass before it's resuscitated and reinvented. And that's a sad reality.

Those were incredible days. Those were incredible days and part of me is nostalgic. Part of me is frightened that we could be nostalgic about something that is that current. I would say ACT UP's major accomplishments are reforming the FDA drug approval process, the main accomplishment, creation of the parallel track and expedited approval and conditional approval and accelerated approval and expanded access programs. The second major effect is forcing industry and the media and the general populace to recognize two things: 1) that health care delivery in this country is a nightmare and needs to be revamped and 2) that patient involvement in decisions made around research and drug development has to be mandated. I think the industry recognizes that. It's still on a company by company basis, but they recognize that we're not guinea pigs. Other effects have been made as well around discrimination around disabled people in general.

Hank Wilson I don't think that AIDS activism has ended. I'm with ACT UP Golden Gate and we're doing good stuff right now with two dozen people in the room. But it's always been partly scream and push and power like muscle. It's always been cerebral and they complement each other. You have to do the homework which is studying the groundwork and then you do the flash. Sometimes you do the flash and, at least if nothing else, it's noted as a footnote in history even if you are getting creamed. But activism means many things. I think it's going to be more complex in the future. It's not going to be just the scream. We've done the scream, you know, the generic scream. We need to fine tune the scream, to be smart and scream specific messages and stuff. That's what's hard. It's not a quick fix. It's going to be a marathon, not a sprint. Although I get off seeing people do a sprint.

Where is the new generation? I'm old compared to you and I know that. I'm like a grandfather at ACT UP. I don't see people in their twenties very often, a few. The other thing, though, is it's always been small numbers of people that have moved the community. It hasn't been thousands; it's always been core groups that are the catalysts for the larger group. That's been through the whole history.

Richard Chavez I think it could have been a little bit more aggressive. I think they should have burned buildings. And that may still happen. You have a community whose struggle and whose goal is to live so dying will not stop them. Changes will not happen unless there is a violent act. We're going to be in front of the State Department whether we have a permit to do it. You just get a bunch of people and you start them sitting down. I don't care since I am going to die anyway, so you lose. I think you will get stuff like that. I advocate that stuff actually. There will be an anger that is coming through people that they will. I'm seeing it from people.

Without a cure in sight

One night at work, conversation wound up on the end of the first generation of AIDS. One man explained: "Go back to the Fall of '93, right after the Berlin AIDS conference, take a look at the obits published in the *BAR*. There were twice the obituaries of PWAs published that fall." The conference had revealed that no research leads were panning out (Rofes, 1996: 3; Kramer, 1993B). "And those PWAs who had lived on hope that a cure was around the corner, who had held faith in science and our institutions, who had been told 'Be Here for the Cure' gave up."

The Halloween night carnival atmosphere in the Castro around the Clinton win in November 1992 seemed like a distant past. The following year's Yokohama meeting produced no better news. "Meeting Lays Bare the Abyss Between AIDS and Its Cure," the *New York Times* reported. "There's obviously some fatigue," Don de Gagne observed. "There's nothing new. I think we have to acknowledge that" (Pollack, 1994).

The Shanti Scandal, marking the demise of the paradigm of the San Francisco Model, broke during spring 1993 (Botkin, 1995). Today, the service net forming the San Francisco Model is crumbling, in need of funds, its volunteers compassion-fatigued with the ongoing epidemic (Lehrman, 1994).

During autumn 1993 ACT UP began what looked like an implosion. Out ran an article titled: "What's Going Down At ACT UP?" when ACT UP DC shut down operations (Chew, 1993). The internal squabbles and such articles as "ACT UP's Split over Issues" continued (Shepnick, 1995).

As all this was going on, the McClintock AIDS Cure Act, H.R. 3310, was introduced to the 103rd Congress thanks to the lobbying of ACT UP. The bill sought to fund a Manhattan type research project to find a cure. Six billion had been appropriated for flood disaster relief that summer; one billion for H.R. 3310 would have ignited the project. H.R. 3310 earned nothing like the coverage of Gays in the Military, the Shanti Scandal, or Whitewater. And, of course, it was lost by November 1994.

Perception problems as political obstacles

What happened to a focus on a cure? It's difficult to say. A series of complex circumstances made taking on HIV disease in Congress particularly contentious. One of the greatest difficulties of forming policies around HIV disease had to do with the fact that HIV has never lacked controversy (Nelson, 1984: 127). During the 1980s, HIV was constructed as a politically contentious issue involving controversial behavior, and the problem never achieved a solution. Human behavior issues are always more difficult to get on the agenda. There is a solid constancy who believe that PWAs are already a politically protected special interest group deviating from the norm of mainstream behavior (Schmitt, 1996). Misconceptions and selective observation prevail to this day.

By 1994 AIDS existed at the withering point of Down's cycle of media attention. The public was tired of hearing about it and people know the answer will be difficult and costly to achieve (Nelson, 1984: 52). "AIDS Still Immune to the Onslaught of Medical Science," Eric Eckholm (1994) wrote on the front page of the *New York Times*. "A reprieve seems farther away than ever." As the abundance of obits in the *BAR*, autumn 1993 reflected, the community lost hope that a cure was ever going to be around the corner. "It's like the light at the end of the tunnel theory," Raoul told me. Other issues hit the forefront. Kingdon (1984) explains "Conditions come to be defined as problems, and have a better chance of rising on the agenda, when we come to believe that we should do something to change them." The operative word here is "believe." Few believed that finding a cure was a possibility (Milano, 1995), so we stopped trying.

"One of the worst things I see happening is that HIV and AIDS are beginning to be treated like some kind of an endemic problem that's just part of the tortured landscape of America," Paul Di Donato, of the San Francisco AIDS Foundation, explained (Mirken, 1994).

Instead of the formation of policies designed to end the epidemic, the Ryan White Care Fund remains in place (Hilts, 1990). Organizations formed under a model of deviance to serve, now regulate and segregate people with AIDS. Hospices were formed to house dying PWAs, keeping them out of sight. Services for PWAs grew contingent on conformity, on social control (Perrow, 1978: 106–7). PWAs were categorized. AIDS Inc. prospered.

PART VII

Institutionalization

TWENTY

AIDS Inc. and the State of Maintenance

As the realization that the epidemic was not going anywhere sunk in, the transition from short- to long-term thinking had a profound effect on AIDS organizations. Groups took the attitude that they needed to jog, not sprint. Activists became dismayed. Disgust with the state of AIDS services pervaded the interviews. Many questioned the intentions of those in the "helping professions." There is a perception that careers and a great deal of money are being made off of PWAs by researchers, health, and service agencies ("Tracking the AIDS Economy," 1995). Without a "magic bullet" cure, AIDS services had became the status quo.

"Maintenance = Death," Cleve Jones proclaimed at the twelfth annual AIDS Candlelight Vigil in 1995. "For every hospice built, bodies will arrive to fill them." By the 1990s, the volunteers who had lined up in force to serve their communities during the mid-1980s watched the very grass-roots organizations they had supported lose sight of their original goals and become bureaucratic monsters. AIDS organizations began putting more effort into courting donors and funds than fighting for their clients. Jane Addams warned about the pitfalls of the "helping profession" (Trattner, 1994). "Most everyone else has fallen into some sort of bureaucracy and it supports an AIDS industry," G'dali reflected. As the "revolution" incorporated, AIDS services and strategies to lobby for a cure stagnated. The San Francisco Model fell into a historic trap of the helping professions.

The bureaucratization of the San Francisco Model follows classic premises of organizational theory. In difficult times, organizations tend to turn to a more centralized authority which is soon followed by disenchantment among staff and clients. Members of such organizations, as we have observed, focus on their own issues as opposed to larger goals. Goal displacement, in which original goals, such as an orientation toward finding a cure, are left behind and replaced with new goals, maintenance of long-term organizations. Survival of such organizations becomes a means in and of itself. Everyone tends to protect his or her own best interests. The Shanti CYOB (Cover Your Own Butt) attitude and unionization of the San Francisco AIDS Foundation follow. Management set rules to control their workers and protect themselves. All of these things distract the organizations from their original goals (Sosin, 1990; Bedian and Zammuto, 1991).

Cleve Jones, like many AIDS activists, would like to see his peers working in the AIDS Industry get back to the Jane Addams form of social activism focusing resources toward ending the epidemic. In taking a macro-look at the San Francisco Model, interviewees talk about the metamorphosis from the grass roots to AIDS Inc.

Cleve Jones   The frightening thing about what's happening now is that there is this emphasis on maintenance. I think that the best and the brightest have died and those that remain are now just struggling to maintain their share of the pie. So in my speeches, when I go out my new slogan is, "Maintenance Equals Death." That there needs to be a new wave of activism that refuses to accept the death of all of us who are infected.

It's been quite strange to watch the power of our community grow as a result of the epidemic. People don't like to admit it, but the fact is gay and lesbian people have much more power in this country than ever before because of the AIDS epidemic, because of the fact that America has come to know its gay and lesbian children as we've gotten sick and died. It's hard to stay in the closet with purple lesions all over your face. And we've discovered the solidarity that does exist within our community, that it was not a transitory thing based on some sexual fad or trend, that it was real and permanent. So now I see an enormous potential that we have. But people don't quite accept the stakes.

It's perfectly clear to me that half of the gay men of my generation and a third of the gay men of your generation are going to die of AIDS unless there's a cure, and that no amount of service providers are going to change that. All of the force of the movement and all of that power right now seems to be directed at housing sick people and feeding sick people and trying to do some education within the guidelines that are allowed. It's very frustrating. If we go on this way everybody is going to die. I don't want to die. I still haven't accepted that I am going to die of AIDS.

Robin Tichane   I think a lot of the focus has been on the individual and Shanti's work as one-on-one. It's important to do that, but the AIDS Foundation and a lot of these places seem to be so focused and so nearsighted. Let's help this individual get through the Social Security paperwork system and it's all months and months and months. Very few people are taking the distance to step back and say "its already 10,000 and it's certainly going to be another 25,000 in this little town."

Hank Wilson This has been a problem in the black community, as groups get institutionalized the industry takes over. There are so many problems in the black community right now. Crack is just destroying them and the black politicians don't always do what they need to do. Service industries perpetuate themselves instead of dealing with problems. We're at that point now where we've gotten institutions. We didn't when we started out. It was all community spirit, community building, not career building. That's the difference. I see that and it hurts.

G'dali Braverman Part of what the evolution of this movement is based on is that some people can't live with the small changes, and they make choices to become part of what I call the AIDS Industry because they think that being on the inside is going to make that change. People struggle to find ways that they feel are going to be more effective. But no one is sitting down to do an assessment and say, "You know what? Maybe it's better to sit down and start from scratch right now."

I tend to have the attitude of "Why assume that anything worked?" We're still in this epidemic; people are still dying. People are clearly still becoming infected. The organizations that have been created have had too limited an impact on public policy, which is a very volatile area that can change with every meeting of the legislature, and no impact on overall treatment. Why not start from scratch and just say, "Everything's failed?" Everything has failed. What do we need to do? Pat ourselves on the back about our successes and try to model a program on them? Those successes are not sufficient enough to warrant modeling something after them.

We, as a microcosm, being the gay-lesbian-AIDS community and its infrastructure, can be dismantled completely. So what we will end up with is lots of PWAs without services and lots of gays and lesbians losing their jobs and having to really re-examine what their true motivation is. Are you here to unionize your job at the San Francisco AIDS Foundation? – which to me is a repulsive idea. I don't think that PWAs working at the AIDS Foundation need to be unionized. Your objective in working at this is to see an end to this disease, not to protect your job. If you need to protect your job, then clearly you're thinking of this as a long-term thing and you're not finding short-term solutions to this epidemic. Big problem there.

Why was ACT UP birthed? Because an option was created, AZT. And it was inaccessible to the masses. This stirred people enough because when a glimmer of hope is there in the mass of confusion then people begin to mobilize. None of that exists now. What we have instead are thousands of superficial glimmers of hope that appease the populace sufficiently to keep them from being activated or mobilized. "That organization will take care of me" or "They're really doing the work. I know they're fighting for me." Those are all false realities. They're band-aids, dog biscuits, whatever.

Raoul Thomas   It's a big money-making venture for a lot of people. I think of how much money gets generated just because of AIDS. It's probably generated billions of dollars. They are kind of making a lot of money off the illness. It's definitely an economic phenomenon.

Hank Wilson   The AIDS Industry, AIDS Inc. supplanted People With AIDS. People With AIDS originally had the AIDS Hotline. People With AIDS had community forums and they did a bunch of stuff. Now the AIDS Foundation has the hotline, has the forums. We lost in this city.

Nancy Lemoins   I'd like to stop the industry of the whole thing, the making money off of people's suffering. Everybody who does a fund-raiser who makes 150 million dollars gives it to the AIDS Foundation. What are they doing with that money? This is why we started this PWA Coalition. If it doesn't get caught up in rhetoric and ego then it might do something. I don't know. I feel pretty disillusioned.

Cleve Jones   Now, I got a problem with AIDS Inc. because AIDS Inc. is based on maintaining the status quo.

Jobs, careers, and a failed hypothesis?

Paul Greenbaum   I think Project Inform has got a very large stake in the HIV hypothesis. I have lobbied a lot to get them to be a little more flexible. They tend to rewrite history from time to time and say, "Oh well, we never really told you to take AZT. We just had early intervention." I thought that was a lot of spin-doctoring and protested to them, "Let's just say we were wrong about this. Everybody was wrong." (*He gives me a copy of "Treatment Strategy, Project Inform Discussion Paper #1, Day One . . . After You've Tested Positive," P4, 5/17/93.*) This AZT statement has been thrown back in everyone's face for years from PI without retrenchment. It's a dangerous postulation, especially in light that uninformed people may use it for other means. *Paul reads:*

> Use of an anti viral should be discussed with your physician as soon as infection by HIV is diagnosed, without waiting for the

appearance of symptomatic illness. The recommendation is to use anti viral medicine anytime the CD4+ count falls below 500. This may be expanded to people with higher counts when other studies are completed. In general, it seems logical to use anti viral medication anytime a person is infected, *perhaps* without regard to CD4+ counts.

Project Inform just won't face the fact, you said anyone who's diagnosed should take AZT, no matter the T-cell number. Why can't they just admit they were wrong?

Yet even with all that I've seen some bureaucratic shenanigans that at times I find a little unsettling. I mean, I am still committed to the goals of the organization, but they do take money from pharmaceutical companies and I don't care what they say, that's going to affect your point of view. The pharmaceutical industry has fairly always been with us. And that money is spent like on going to Berlin or Amsterdam [for AIDS conferences]. I really think it could be better spent around the office providing direct services instead of supporting a little cadre of careerists, which is what we have there now. But, whether I like it or not, PI is going to be part of my life.

The state of maintenance

Service groups are required to follow certain stipulations to receive funds. These conditions often stifle the freedom of those accessing the services. Per, Hugo, Darnell, Cynora and Yvonne discuss the state of AIDS services.

Darnell Davis I moved twice in a two-month period. Do you know how exhausted I am? I went to the people running the building I just moved out of, I says, "Look, my life is wonderful; I've everything on track. I have a one-room apartment, but my concern is maintaining my home." What did they do? The first thing they fucked with is my God damned home. So I moved out. I'd rather sit and die by myself, in my own shit, than to allow some of these people to take care of me.

I was under the impression that I was moving into a building that was there for HIV people who needed help with low-income housing. I agreed to come in there and pay low rent. I did not agree to any other program. I didn't need a caseworker. I was not aware that I had people policing me every day or that someone could come to my house at the age of 35 and say, "You can't have guests, you're on house restriction." I don't need that shit! When you take away the people that love you, deny them access to me, then you take away a lot from me. Then you make me totally dependent on you, and that means you can rub me anyway you want. So that means that I have to sit down and say, "Yes, yes, yes," when I say, "No, no, no." In other words: "Fuck you. You don't live here. I do. You go home and you entertain your guests and you have dinner. I can't. What? Because you've agreed to give me low-income housing." If that's the price to pay for low-income housing, then it's no longer helping the people.

The false facade is that they are here to help people. When my T-cell drops, my stress level skyrockets; that's not helping. In a two-month period, I lost more weight and sleep and gained more stress than I have over the whole fucking year that my lover died. That's pathetic. If they were able to do that to me, can you imagine what would happen to someone that isn't as strong as I am?

I was treated like I was brought in there off the street. In one meeting, I says, "Oh, I went to visit my nieces." She says, "It must be nice to finally have an address!" Excuse me? I had an address before I got here. That just showed me where her head was. You think about these things and wonder how deep does this attitude in the organization run? You're dealing with people's emotions at a point in their lives where their self-esteem is very low, their tolerance of pain is very low. And you have someone dishing out that much pain, it goes deep.

I was able to move out. I'm going to die the same way I live, with pride and dignity, and you can't have that. And that's what they strip. You take that pride, dignity and self-respect away, we just have a hollow shell. We have people walking around scared; these are adults, they're having the roughest time of their lives. Faced with something that a lot of people have no perception of what these people are feeling, mentally and physically. And they're taking away from them the last little thing that they have left in their heart. If they're just going to take that away, who the fuck wants to live?

Hugo Manzo   After that first Shanti House, I moved to the concentration camp in which I am living now. Concentration camp, why do I say that? One of my friends says every time he goes to visit me he thinks he's entering a place where people are being held hostage instead of a place where people are being helped. It's mostly red tape I think, and not really wanting to really help. Instead it's just making a name by showing the community, "This is what we are doing for PWAs." They're doing it for themselves, not for us.

How would I do if I were to run the place? Well, first of all I would become involved in doing more fund-raising for the building itself because it needs a lot of maintenance. Secondly, I would take away a lot of the rules that they have. I would fight the government around money being given under strict conditions which cause these rules. If you make money the government can take away your funds. It takes away the dignity of the persons. I would make it very different. I would be on the side of the clients, not on the side of the government. After a long time people tend to forget why they really started working and they become bureaucrats and not helpers.

I am sad that they have used AIDS, this disease, to make money, to make a political career out of it. The only agency that I give an A+ is the AIDS Emergency Fund, the very agency that does not pay any staff but two or three; the rest are volunteers and help clients directly. If we have more agencies like that, the government would not have to spend so much money. 'Cause most of the money that the government gives to the AIDS epidemic is not going to the people. It's blocked by the bureaucrats in the middle. They have made an industry out of AIDS and they don't let the people receive the money. That needs to be changed. Don't say you are going to help because that's playing with God's principles. When you play with God's laws you have come onto a very dangerous ground.

Goal displacement

Per Eidspjeld I went away for two months and came back and wanted to go see the people that I knew there [in an HIV recreation program]. Here I was standing in their lobby and they wouldn't let me in to say "Hi" because they changed their policy. Some insurance company took over so they had to have a letter, and then they said, "Now, you have to be here at least three times a week. You have to." I am not going to commit myself to that just because of some policy. I never went back. I actually got disappointed with the whole thing. It was helpful to me to go there and meet other people and have a meal with them, network with these people. I have a problem with all these conformed organizations. If you're going to look into all the AIDS organizations in San Francisco, you wouldn't have time to do anything else.

Cynora Jones Fuck these organizations about. I'm sorry I'm using that real freely, but that's the way I feel about a lot of the referral sources. It's that people have other fucking agendas. "I have something else that I would rather do because then I'll be this person in this community with this much clout." You run into that. I'm so sick of other people telling us what we need. They have councils they set themselves on. I'm tired of being the poor little woman with AIDS. I got to depend on you for every mother-fucking thing.

Yvonne Knuckles They need to put more people out in the field, outreach, talking to find these people and talk out in open places instead of sitting in offices and letting people know where the help is, someone out there telling 'em where to get help. Go in these places you're afraid to go in. That's where the people are with it.

The need for consolidation

Cleve Jones When I ran for office here two years ago, one of my campaign themes was the need to centralize and consolidate AIDS services, which I see as now beginning to be addressed. We've got a situation now in which too much money is going into administrative costs. If you've got a hundred agencies, there's actually more than a hundred agencies in San Francisco alone, providing services to PWAs. And every one of them has an executive director, a development director, a media coordinator, and a volunteer coordinator. Can we consolidate some of these? Can there be one centralized volunteer intake and training process, for example?

Jay Segal Lots of it has got to be consolidated, especially right now at this minute because we just lost $220,000 from our San Francisco AIDS budget. Part of what Project Inform has been telling the government, and it doesn't apply to them because I've tried to do it, is: the reason the government is failing is that we have 318 AIDS organizations all doing the same thing differently at the same time, splitting the money up 318 ways. If we had one project at a time and we took all 318 people and they did their expertise on that particular project and we didn't stop that project until we got it done, it would work. But PI who is doing 318 different things at once, will not do that same thing themselves. I say to them, "If you do this yourself and it works on this scatterbrained organization, it should be that much easier to sell to the government or the city bureaucracies. Look, it worked for us, try it." It makes sense to me 'cause there's a lot of brains out there and a lot of people who aggressively want to get this thing. Their efforts are wasted because there is just so much going on at the same time. Even if somebody came up with a cure, it would get blurred in the mirror and nobody would see it. There's still the question of "If we got a cure how would we get it to the people?"

The next wave

The epidemic is evolving, changing faces, and ultimately becoming more intertwined with American poverty. Today, HIV death rates and the probabilities of dying from HIV are substantially higher among blacks than among whites. Gay men continue to get sick (Gross, 1993; Odets, 1995). Rates of infection never slowed (Rofes, 1996: 173–8). There was a 13 percent increase in AIDS deaths among black men in 1994, the last year for which such numbers are available. AIDS caused at least one of every three deaths among black men aged twenty-five to forty-four (Hilts, 1996A). The evolving face of the epidemic proved extremely difficult for the bureaucracies of AIDS Inc. to handle.

Cleve Jones   One of the most unfortunate things that has happened is that, at least in San Francisco and elsewhere, various communities, particularly communities of color and women, weren't being served appropriately by the agencies that were created mainly by men like myself, middle-class background, white, urban gay men. As the epidemic has changed and grown, it is not always appropriate for these organizations to be run by white, middle-class, urban, gay men. So a lot these agencies serving, particularly people of color, set up their own independent agencies. While they were well motivated, I don't think it's really solved the problem they were trying to address. Instead they have become further marginalized and as the funding opportunities have failed to expand with the epidemic, there's enormous competition between groups.

Another problem has been that many of the agencies that were set up by gay people were set up by people like myself who did not have backgrounds in public health but in political activism and were interested in our little turf wars. But the most fundamental change that's happened is that you now have agencies like Gay Men's Health Crisis where a majority of their clients are not gay men. This puts us all through all sorts of changes because, of course, the gay community has this great sense of ownership of the disease and the agencies that were created to fight it. They are often the bases of political power for activists within our community. That's not right or wrong, it's just the way it is. So, things have got to change.

242

Ronnie Ashley It was real funny 'cause I had a volunteer once turn around and tell me, literally turn around and cuss me and read me and told me that he didn't want to work with any other population and didn't want to work with "Those people." He only wanted to work with gay white men and gay white men only, and that he was sick and tired of the agency oppressing gay white men blah, blah, blah, blah, blah, blah. It was like, "You know what, time out for a second, because you insult me as an Indian, as a gay man and as a person of color."

Hugo Manzo I wish that all the AIDS agencies, Shanti Project, Latino AIDS Project and all the other little agencies will disappear. We need new structures. We definitely need new structures. Why? Because the structures that we have for the AIDS agencies are based on gay people. Is that wrong? No, it's not wrong, but it's not only gay people that are getting infected. It's everyone. So we need to change the structures so that we can serve better. That's what the ongoing problem has been.

We're still caught up in thinking AIDS is a gay disease and we don't want to change that. We show that by not changing the strategies of helping or changing the structures of the agencies that help people.

Ronnie Ashley The figures in 1995 from the CDC out of Florida, everybody is freaked out because 25 percent of their AIDS cases are coming out of the elderly community. You got Grandma and Grandpa, they got full-blown AIDS and everybody's freaked. Well why? they're not a high-risk community; they're not doing drugs but they're fucking. Hello, (*laughs*) if you are having unprotected sex, you are at high risk, plain and simple. I don't give a fuck who you are. And you could carry that Bible from here to hell, child, 'cause that's where you're going to end up if you don't snap and realize.

As the demographics of the epidemic change, HIV's impact on the mortality of black Americans is likely to increase (McDaniel and London, 1995). And the new wave of HIV will produce new stories.

Cynora Jones The epidemic that's beginning to get unveiled here in the East Bay is going to blow people's minds. I see a big change. I was doing outreach, passing out condoms on 14th Street in Oakland. I had one guy tell me, who already had AIDS, "Why do I need to use a condom? I'm already infected." Why would the person want to perpetuate their life if they already think that everybody who gets this disease is going to die from it anyway? There's no education. There's no hope. We can't fight. We can't live. We won't be here long enough to make this disease die. What difference does it make?

243

Yvonne Knuckles This one guy came up to me about six months ago and told me he had the virus, he be down there, right? He wanted to ask me, do I think this other girl he had been with had it. I said, "I don't know how you got it but you shoulda used a condom." You know you're having all these different people, picking up all these young girls. You're having sex with them. Now he's walking around, trying to find out, wondering which one he got it from. I said, "Well, you will probably never know that. Now you know that you should've used a condom, right?" So we're talking now. He was the one who was, "I'm not ever going to do this or put a condom on."

Long-term problems and pieces of the pie

Cleve Jones I am very concerned that there is this great focus on maintaining our share of the Ryan White pie. I was at this conference recently where I overheard people over at the next table celebrating the fact that their city had now been added to the list of Title One cities and so there were going to be more job opportunities for them. I don't begrudge anybody getting paid to do this; I get paid for what I do. But we need to recognize that we are part of an industry. My little personal joke is, "God, if they find a cure I'm going to have to find a real job." AIDS Inc. doesn't worry me. What worries me is the attitudes of the people who work for AIDS Inc. Are they going to fight for a cure?

AIDS in context

I think there has to be a whole break and we have to say, (*begins hitting the table*) "No, we are not gonna just build more fucking hospices! We are going to find a God damned cure and we are going to save the people that are infected."

Raoul Thomas It's really an emergency, all alarm bells have gone off. A fire has broken out; now it's time to put it out. It's a meltdown. It really is.

Cleve Jones And I think Larry [Kramer] said years ago, maybe y'all ought to shut down and let the bodies stack out in the streets. Let people see what the hell is going on here. I said it last night at the Candlelight March. I said, "I want to talk to all the caregivers out there. I know that most of you are caregivers out there either in your own homes or the agencies and organizations. I know you feed the hungry, and clothe the naked, and

AIDS INC. AND THE STATE OF MAINTENANCE

shelter the homeless, and dispel ignorance. None of that and none of these candles and none of these quilts is going to save my life. I want you to save my life. I don't want to die." I'm going to get the service providers, I want them to push the absolute limit of their 501(C3) status (*tax exemption status for non-profit organizations*). How many meals are delivered in this country every day to home-bound people with AIDS? Every one of those meals should have a pre-addressed envelope to that person's Congress member. How many people are going through intake interviews every day in every city and town in this country right now? People down there (*directed at myself as a staff member of an AIDS agency*) tell them that whether they live or die is going to depend on the congressional allocations for research.

Marching is worthless except it makes you feel good. How many of those people there, there were about 5000 people there last night, I betcha if you asked, "How many of you really have sat down and put pen to paper in the last year to a member of Congress?" maybe a dozen people would raise their hands. It's very frustrating.

Another thing I find frustrating is that the politicized activists throw around this terrible burden of cynicism. I had lunch here at this restaurant two weeks ago with Larry Kramer and Martin Delanney and Mike Shriver. They are much more cynical than I am. I think part of it is that I get out into America all the time. I'm going to little towns and big cities every day. I think there is an incredible reservoir of good will and intelligence out there and that the American public is not hysterical about AIDS any more. Most of them are not full of hatred and most of them have learned that they have a gay person in their family. I really think that's where the country's at. And that's backed up by a whole lot of those surveys so that even the right-wingers begin to splinter and divide over these issues. So you've got these activists who are so cynical. You've got gay people who do not want to give up ownership of the disease.

The same old education void

Right now every fucking school board in the country has some right-wing asshole on there whose gonna censor what the kids get. It's difficult to walk through the city and not see a bus poster about AIDS. It's maddening to me and I go to places where there is no AIDS education and then, you know, these dumb kids waking up, realizing they're queer in Duluth and Des Moines and Dubuque and getting on the Greyhound and coming out here. They're clueless and they're broke and often they're alcoholic and drug-addicted and abused. This is where I get sad again because I believed that your generation of gay kids would grow up not experiencing the kind of self-hatred that my generation experienced. I thought that that would change forever, yet it appears that it has not. And when you read the focus group reports of these interviews, from the AIDS Foundation, with these under twenty-one-year-olds who are infected, it's heartbreaking. They say all the love in the community is going to people with AIDS; all gay people have to die; this is my destiny. It was just like this thing I saw interviewing black women, black girls with babies. They're asking these children, "Why did you have children?" "Well, it was the only way I could get somebody to love me." I hate to use the little buzz words of the day, but it's all about self-esteem and it breaks my heart to see there are so many gay kids growing up with the same bullshit. I know what their lives are going to be like. I know they're gonna be strung out on drugs or alcohol or dead from AIDS very soon. So the struggle continues and lives are still at stake.

Ronnie Ashley Hello! The United States needs to get up off its ass and learn something from Amsterdam and from Switzerland where they have the lowest IV drug use anywhere, the lowest in AIDS-infected anywhere. Why? Because the shit's legal. Yes, they are getting clean needles. Yes, they are getting the information. That's another thing, how do you turn around and teach anal retentive America about safe sex? What is safe sex? It's a hell of a lot more than just putting on a fucking condom. How the hell are you going to straight out and forwardly talk about what men and men do together, what women do together? People don't want to hear about how they're getting whipped and how they're getting butt fucked and how there are clit piercings and so on and so forth. We can't talk about that shit. Yet at the same time they can't handle it when the priest is blowing up someone's skirt. People are so fucking anal retentive about their sexuality, they don't got a fucking clue.

Jesse Helms sitting up there on the God damned floor of the House waving this fucking pamphlet talking about: "You read this shit, you're gonna become queer." Well, motherfucker, who are you fucking and what's his name? Because it's obvious you read it. (*Chuckles.*) "It's too blunt for our children to read . . ." I've been fucking around since I was a ten-year-old child and believe me, I knew I was playing. We all know that we are playing. We all know that we are going to touch ourselves and, no Grandma, we ain't going blind (see Neff, 1996).

Stonewall and beyond

Almost every PWA I talked to responded that they wished there was more of a focus on finding a cure as opposed to a social service model. Interviewees look at first-generation AIDS in the context of Stonewall.

Hank Wilson The other challenge is, if people are homophobic and they vote against us, we still can move them. We still can make progress. If homophobia is on a scale from 1 to 40 and we can move people to 16, where they started at 6, that's progress, even though they vote against us. To fight the fight is to win, even when we lose. That sounds like a contradiction but it's not. We've got more people now than we ever have and that's because of AIDS. That's the silver lining. It's brought people out of the closet. We're also perceived by many people as a caring community, not just a sexual community.

Cleve Jones I'm frustrated with AIDS Inc. but I think you have to separate that out from Gay and Lesbian Liberation. Unlike other social movements, especially movements of economically oppressed people, Gay and Lesbian Liberation is about personal liberation. It's about individuals deciding to live their lives openly and honestly and it is a great deal about love and a need for relationships.

But I think the reason why we have advanced so far in the gay struggle over the last ten years is because so many men and women found themselves confronted in some way in their lives by this virus and were forced to take a stand, were forced to come out, were forced to care for people and to realize that the times required them to act. I still get blown away when I see 300,000 people at Gay Pride Marches. It's interesting that out of all the social movements born in the late '60s, there's only one that still has the power to bring hundreds of thousands out on the streets on a regular basis.

I just think, I was a Gay Liberationist first, I was a Gay Liberationist for ten years before the epidemic, and right now we're under assault on all these different fronts. There's gonna be big battles about gays in the military, the right to marriage, domestic partners, custody, job discrimination, hate crime. In each of these struggles people are going to suffer and people are going to lose their children, and their families and people are going to be beaten and killed, but when you add it all up, even all together, the total pales in significance compared to the toll that AIDS is going to take on our people. So for me it's very clear that in the whole range of issues facing gay and lesbian people, this remains the number one issue, and under the whole range of issues under the heading AIDS, research for a cure has to be a number one priority there. That's sort of where I'm at now, after being sick last year, kind of losing health for a while. I feel a little bit of hope again.

Hank Wilson   I am very proud of my community. We responded. We created institutions that are now institutionalized. At the beginning they weren't on the map. We took care of ourselves. We took care of each other and that feels real good. However flawed we are, like all of these things, like the Shanti Model and all that, we did it. It came from real energy. To me, that's incredible. It's something that no one can take away from us, no matter how it plays out.

PART VIII

Parting Glances

TWENTY-ONE

Ghosts Walking Down Castro Street

At the Shanti House on Market Street, when people die, families usually donate their books to the building library. Books are difficult to transfer. Between stacks of 12-Step workbooks, mysteries, a Marilyn Monroe biography and a copy of *Gone With the Wind*, a stained green hardback sits. The cloth holding the binding is peeling. The book appears to have been doused with water at one point. The words on the cover, barely legible with wear, read, "And the Band Played On – Randy Shilts." Diligently applied Scotch tape holds the hard white top cover onto the green binding. Beneath the tape one reads two words, a name written in blue ink, perhaps that of the previous owner whose copy had been donated to the library. God knows how many PWAs' hands the beaten-up first edition has passed through, informed before they shuffled off this mortal coil themselves, like the original owner. They're gone; Randy Shilts is gone; most of those Randy Shilts interviewed for the text are gone. Most of the Stonewall Generation, most of the '70s migrants to the Castro are gone. Over 100 people died at Shanti House during my two years there who might have picked up the old volume with a slight tint of mildew. Like every author of an AIDS book, I read *And the Band Played On* first, learned about the history of Market Street where we worked, watched Gay Pride, AIDS Candlelight, 49er Superbowl and Halloween cavalcades pass. Shilts informed us about the 1978 Gay Pride Parade on Market which Cleve led, galvanizing the crowd against the Briggs Initiative and then the two years later when he sat with Anne Kronenberg on the Ferris Wheel at Gay Parade 1980, wondering what the future held in store during the last Gay Pride Parade of the Before Period.

Leaves and sheets of newspaper accumulate in the front door area of the lobby on Market as people move in and out all day. The first time anyone died during my tenure, a gust of wind grabbed one of those newspaper pages, perhaps from an old *Bay Area Reporter* with its weekly list of obits from the plague. The page flew out the front door along with a few leaves, through the August air out onto Market Street. Rob was gone. People seldom talk about the folks who have died at Shanti House.

We don't know where they are or what to make of it. "When I walk down Castro Street, I'm accompanied by ghosts, but always very proud," Cleve Jones reflected in a 1990 interview (Fernandez, 1991). Up Market to Castro, the same route he had led his processions over the last twenty years, Cleve met me for lunch at the Patio Café. I opened the 1987 copy of *And the Band Played On* from the building, wanting to know where Cleve was at, eight years later. I wanted Cleve's words, Cleve's response to the epic of his life Randy Shilts had chronicled through over two volumes and left behind, uncompleted. The now salt-and-pepper-haired, slightly embarrassed Cleve Jones pleaded, "Lower your voice." I read from the epilogue recalling a 1987 White House demonstration and his thoughts:

> Much of what he had once dreamed for would not come to pass; Cleve accepted that now. In years past, Cleve and the other citizens of Castro Street had looked ahead to a time when they had rooted out prejudice against gay people altogether and healed the lives that the prejudice had scarred. They might be old men by then, but they would be able to entertain each other with reminiscences of the old days when they had all believed they could change the world, and know that to a certain extent, they had. Many of those people are dead now, and Cleve accepted that most of his friends would be dead before they reached anything near old age.
>
> What hadn't changed for Cleve was the dream itself; what they had fought for, what Harvey Milk had died for, was fundamentally right, Cleve thought. It had been a fight for acceptance and equality, against ignorance and fear. It was that fight that had brought Cleve to Washington on this day.
>
> The number of AIDS cases measured the shame of the nation, he believed. The United States, the one nation with the knowledge, the resources, and the institutions to respond to the epidemic, had failed. And it had failed because of ignorance and fear, prejudice and rejection. The story of the AIDS epidemic was that simple, Cleve felt; it was a story of bigotry and what it could do to a nation.
>
> The legacy of the nation's shame could be read in the faces that Cleve always carried in his memory, the faces of the dead. Cleve could see those faces now as he led the chant at the wrought iron gates of the White House: "Shame. Shame. Shame." Tears streamed down his cheeks as he raised his fist toward the Oval Office. He saw Simon Guzman and Bobbi Campbell . . . (pp. 600–1)

"Stop," Cleve whispered in a broken voice, from across the small table, a red teary face before the final line, "And, of course, he saw Bill Kraus."

"Its tough, I got that way when I read it."

"I miss Randy. You know during the floods they brought in the helicopters to Gernville Cemetery and they all landed right on Randy," Cleve laughed with a sigh of catharsis.

"That was eight years ago. What about those dreams? How does one keep on living with those dreams?"

Cleve Jones Well, they're happening baby. It's still going on. It's still happening. We're still doing it. I'm proud of it. It was all my idea and I started the whole thing. (*Laughing.*) Last year, I gave up. Last year I was really depressed. But I think even in the worst of the depression, what I was sad about was that I wasn't going to get to watch it tomorrow. There's a very personal sort of sense of feeling ripped off that I wasn't going to be able to be an old man and sit around and tell these stories. And I very much wanted that, but I am feeling better now. I've been feeling really hopeful the last almost six months now about being able to keep fighting again. I feel sort of pissed off that I cannot express very well. I'm not a very religious person but I think that there are clues out there and I do believe in good and evil. I believe that what we are doing is good, that the lessons we're learning from the epidemic transcend the epidemic, that it's about sanctity of life, sanctity of love. I just feel very much like I've been blessed and allowed to work with some of the most incredible people and that we have touched millions of lives and we changed lives. It's not rhetoric. I know that to be true. I really know it to be true. Just while I was waiting to meet you walking up and down this street, I had about twenty people just come up and say, "Gosh it's really good to see you alive." I just get this sense that there is a continuity and that there is a promenade. Good people keep trying to make the world better, try to stop fighting and try to teach people to love each other. In a weird way, the epidemic has advanced that understanding, at a terrible cost; I know I'm probably not going to make it. I still feel really amazed and privileged to be experiencing all this.

When I was a little boy, my parents were sort of intellectuals. I never got much of an education myself. My parents were both college professors. But I used to read all these books. I just felt, I want to do something with my life. I don't want to have a job and family. I want to do something with my life, how?

So last night actually turned out to be a good night, twelve years after Fighting For Our Lives (the first AIDS Candlelight Vigil; Cleve came up with the title for the banner carried in 1983 proclaiming those words). "Tell me about last night?"

Last night was nice because I haven't been to an event like that in San Francisco in over two years and a lot of my friends thought I was dead, I think. It was just very good to see everybody that's not dead. And then to remember, I think the first time I marched down Market Street was '73, '72, all the Harvey Milk marches and the big protest marches. It's just I've been doing it for twenty-something years.

I would like to be remembered as a fairly ordinary person of average intelligence and good humor who did help. I think I have helped create some rituals that are going to be really enduring. Candlelight Marches, I started that, the rainbow flag, a whole range of stuff. These have been things that bind people together, better than rhetoric, better than ideology, and that's what I have done.

White nights and ascending shadows

The White Night Riot – it was pivotal. I don't know what I remember and what I've made up and what I'm repeating that other people have told me. But when I think back on the '70s, it was so new. It was just so new. We'd never done this before. We'd never had the courage to do it before. It seemed like it was just the other day when I was saying to myself, where did all these people come from? Can they really all be homosexuals? There was all this awareness growing up in the cities, in the small towns, all over the place. I was living in Tempe, Arizona when I was first exposed to the notion of the gay community, a gay movement that was not just furtive meetings in bathrooms or parks or dark bars. That was brand-fucking new. Then there was this mass immigration, all of a sudden, right about '75, flooding into the city and forming these communities. Then I think, there was one very important time, and that was Harvey Milk, at least in San Francisco. The time of Harvey Milk was where it all gelled. The riot was a declaration of existence. We are here; we have come this far and no, we will not ever allow you to turn back the clock. It's such a weird little twist of fate that right at that point, as we got there then . . . I mean I thought when Harvey Milk got killed, what could happen next? What could possibly? Well, *(chuckles)* talk to me now, you know, Harvey Milk, one dead, big deal, talk about a million dead.

The ghost dance continues

That's one of my favorite things. I talk about the ghost dance all the time. I think the closest thing we have to that is the unfolding of the quilt, that ritual. It's very simple, but people dress in white and do this very choreographed thing of unfolding it. And it's repeated almost every day somewhere in the world.

I throw Art's untitled poem in front of Cleve's face:

SIOUX DREAMED
   THE GHOST DANCE

OUT OF HOPE AND GRIEF

BELIEVING THEY COULD
   DANCE BACK
   THEIR DEAD
   THE WARRIOR
   THE BUFFALO

THE COMMUNION
OF LIVING AND DEAD
WAS   FOR SOME
   TOO FRIGHTENING
    (I.E. POWERFUL)

THE FIRST GROUP
   WAS DISPERSED
    (I.E. MASSACRED)

BUT THE DANCE CONTINUES.

PERHAPS WE NEED A NEW GHOST DANCE
A DANCE FOR THE JEWS
A DANCE FOR THE WITCHES
A DANCE FOR THE GAY MEN
A DANCE FOR COMMUNION AND HOPE

I WOULD HAVE IT BE FRIGHTENING.

Yeah, I would have it be frightening too. I talk about it (*the Ghost Dance*) a lot. I hope that it's not a complete rehearsal. I don't think that it is.

Final words and visions

Some concluded with responses to the question, "If a historian from another era came back to Earth to ask about the first generation of the AIDS epidemic, what was it? What was the first generation like, what happened? What would you tell him or her?" I asked every interviewee for final words. Some expressed gratefulness and contemplated the future or if there was even a point; others cut things short. "I don't know, fuck it. Now those are words of wisdom," Brad contributed with a smile and a puff of his cig. Others recalled their own histories and envisioned another ghost dance.

Raoul Thomas   I almost look at it like it's an alien organism visiting from another place in the universe to teach us, but it all involves tragedy. I don't see that too much other stuff comes out of AIDS. The whole thing around AIDS and children, it's all just tragedy to me. To tell you the truth, I wish we weren't doing this. It's like a bad dream really.

Paul Greenbaum   Every group has its particular challenge. For my father it was WW I; for myself it is a disease. But everybody dies.

Marija Mrdjenovic   Well, right now, I really didn't realize this, but I am one of the few women who will talk about AIDS and talk about it in great detail. I'm also not sitting here saying "Government is really wrong," and "This is really wrong." I know what's wrong about this situation. There's a great deal of greed here; there is a great deal of resistance here, that is historical. I guess what I need to see is more changes. If I could change the minds of doctors and get them to change the minds of pharmaceutical companies on what is the right way to treat a patient and what isn't. Right now, it's really a puppet-master situation. If I could get out there and not only let women know that they can challenge the situation, that is what I'd like to do. I'd like them to know that I don't intend to just sit here and die. And I think a lot of the well-meaning artists still think that people will just sit down and die. I'm just not going to be one of them. (*Laughs.*)

Postscript: After the interview, I asked Marija if she would be willing to have her picture taken for the book. She said that would be fine. So, a month later I called and left a couple of messages about setting up a time for the photo shoot and didn't hear back from her. One night at work, I picked up my messages and there was one from Marija's husband: "Ben, I am sorry I didn't get back to you earlier. I don't know how to say this, and I hate to say this on the machine, but Marija died. She went home to visit her mother, got sick and never came out of it."

Richard Chavez People are living on the streets with AIDS; people are living on the streets, period. We're going to have to pay for that as a country, as a consciousness. Something wrong will happen, karma, I guess. And we're already seeing it. We're not living in a country of wealth any more. I think we're paying. Society is moving from civilized to uncivilized. The shadow of our country is coming through, starting to raise its ugly head.

G'dali Braverman I think that I will die and another twenty to thirty years of this epidemic will continue. I think that the next one to two generations of gays and lesbians will be decimated, gay men, not really lesbians. I think we'll lose most of those generations. I think that the community will take another ten years to reorganize and begin looking at how to really re-confront this issue, AIDS.

The first generation was . . .

Nancy Lemoins I think it's like at the beginning of any movement, it had a lot of heart. The way that communities came together, some faster than others, in proportion to the need was pretty amazing. It's never going to be like this again. I think it's like AIDS in Africa; when really huge amounts of people get it, it stops being personal. That's why I want to do art so it stays personal on some level.

Hazel Betsey The first generation of AIDS was a time when people were dropping like flies. People were just dying. It seemed like people got diagnosed and died the next week. But what was happening back then was nobody knew they had it and by the time they found out they had it, it was too late. They already had KS or they already had PCP. There were no preventive measures for PCP. So they got this pneumonia and they died. There was no Septra, no this, no that. I have a friend who was down at San Francisco General Hospital that saw doctors freaking out, families freaking out. People were afraid to have sex for a while. I saw other people committing suicide. There was fear everywhere, fear of people finding out that their kids were gay, "Don't tell me that, you're going to get AIDS," fear of children who got infected through other ways. (*Laughs.*) It was scary, terrifying, but it wasn't something that I was going to get.

Brad Sherbert It was deadly, because when people first started getting sick they very seldom lasted more than six months. It was just massive paranoia everywhere, back in the early '80s, even among the gay community.

Robin Tichane I have every confidence that in 50 to 500 years, because of my use of conservation techniques, my stuff is going to be around and communicating to future generations. This was what AIDS was like and the experience of it in the late twentieth century.

John Cailleau As a community or as members of this village population, we have had to go from big muscles and flat stomachs and being twenty- and thirty-something to getting old and dying and walking with canes. You look at the Castro now and it's not that unusual to see somebody with the thinness of wasting disease who is walking on the arm of a friend, and some of these super bodies that have just shrunk on the inside. It is as much a statement of the strength and character of the gay community that we have managed to survive and continue to incorporate them into the community rather than pushing them out onto an ice float to die. But what also has happened, now that the dream landscape of Castro and the San Francisco of the '70s disappeared, probably not to return within our lifetimes, many people have since said screw it and moved to Seattle or back home. They disappear and die. Most of my close gay friends have, for the most part, died or moved. There is a bond among gay men and some lesbians because we had to grow up in this culture that said who we were is not OK. We weren't supposed to be who we are, and with that shared experience there was a natural bonding. AIDS has not destroyed the bonding, but it's displaced the people and the bodies.

Hugo Manzo I am very tired. I have had HIV for seven years. That is a long time. A lot of people think I look healthy and fine but they don't know how sick I really am inside. My body is like a shiny red apple with worms running through, eating away at it. I know it's ready to start decaying. If I were to die tonight, tomorrow, it would be the happiest day of my life. Sometimes I wish I would.

Robert Boulanget Now we live a little bit more. It's heavier but a different kind of heavy. It's more the real thing. I keep saying to this friend of mine that I'm blessed. It's kind of weird to say you are blessed because you have AIDS, but at least I know I've got my AIDS. I figure that the whole world's got AIDS in a way. Everybody has some sort of AIDS. They all have to put up with something and there's nothing worse than AIDS. The young girl who is kidnapped and molested, I mean she's got AIDS for life. It's just as bad for her as for me to know that I may die next week or may get real sick tomorrow. So I can't say that I'm worse off than they are. It's just all relative. It's a disease that the world has. The United States has got AIDS in a way, being eaten up at the core by something. This is like an illusion. You know you are surrounded by beauty here. I guess it takes the roughness of reality away and creates like a screen that you look at. It's good, although I keep thinking all of our days are counted, if not that, for something else. My God, some animals and some plants live an hour. So whatever it is we are here for, no matter how long it takes, when you get it done, you get it done.

Cities crumble

Jay Segal There's a whole age group that seems to be missing, that's my age group in the forties. This is when you peter out. I've seen all my friends peter out. That's why I don't understand what's happened to me. I'm getting healthy. I'm getting better.

Robin Tichane The biggest social change in my life in the period of my diagnosis has been massive loss to AIDS of my companions and friends. In 1982, there were an estimated 40,000 gay men in San Francisco between the ages of twenty-five and fifty. By 1992, virtually all of the 10,000 deaths from AIDS in San Francisco came from this group.

When I look back

Hank Wilson I see some incredibly strong people who aren't here. I have a lot of sadness. I have people that I used to call up at night and we would bullshit and talk. I don't have people like that now. That was fun and I still remember that. I still value that. They are a strength. I think we were very lucky. I've been very lucky. I've worked with some incredible people. I think at one time we magnetized a lot of people who came here who had a lot of vision and we fed on each other's energy. I remember a group of people who moved this community forward who didn't have personal agendas, who asked the hard questions when they needed to be asked, who were not career people. They weren't career politicians or career in the industry. That really helped. It helped. It used to be that I would go to a community meeting and I would look around and I would see two or three honest ethical people in there. It didn't matter, you knew if they were present. I still think of them when I go to a meeting and I want to be powerful or do what's right even if it's not popular. They're my role models.

We gave each other support and not before the meeting. We're at the right place at the right time to make history and we have been since the '70s and we still are. This is what's been very special about San Francisco. I still feel like that. I just have to get renewed, which still happens. I hope for continuity, but right now we have a new generation and they don't even know what we did.

Dan Vojir I straddled a time that was very very good. When I was coming out there were places that were both gay and straight or they turned gay after a certain time. I'm really appreciative that I could see the time from the '60s to the early '70s when things were still so tight that it was just really weird to be gay, really outcasts. You can't imagine what we had to go through back then. I wouldn't be in a different time slot in the century, I'm very appreciative of when I was born. I stick to my premise, go back to *The Group*, to the ones who took the government jobs who never got out of Illinois. For every one of them, I've lived three lives, three of their lives.

The obits

John Cailleau Most of my friends have already died. I read the *BAR* now and I don't know anybody. I don't even recognize the faces. They're all gone. It's all of these people from the period I'm talking about, late '70s and early '80s, who are dead now. All those associates from the early '80s and late '70s are gone. It moves me just to think about it. Now when I read the obits I don't know anyone who has died that week because everybody I know died months, or years, ago. There's two kinds of obits, those that I had personal contact with somewhere in my life here in the city, like former roommates or people who were former customers or fabric printers. Then there were the people who were just the anonymous faces who I would see at the parties and on the streets and who I never really knew. I'd open up *BAR* and there was this face, turned out to be so and so and so and so. So many faces of people I used to see around all the time who I never really knew, those faces whose I only got to know when they are gone. The first time that I learned that that guy with the big knuckles and a crew cut and a mustache was Joe So and So from such and such a town. He was just what I would call one of the village people. Just the other day I was reading the *BAR* and I saw an ad for a wheelchair and leather chaps. As far as I'm concerned, that tells it all. If I talk about it, it begins to get to me. I'm really not back from that. (*Face fogs.*) I'm not surprised by my reaction. It is a powerful feeling. It's all the little griefs that never were big enough to get expressed at the time. It's like all the sexual energy that built up and built up.

Dealing with HIV is the final polishing of a person's soul. You take a bunch of rough stones, you put them in the tumbler. They're just rocks when they go in. You run them for a few years and they turn out to be polished and beautiful. If a person can make it and live in the world with AIDS or HIV and meet the challenges inherent in that, which in my case is patience, then if I die, so be it. I go into the great cosmic pool of consciousness.

I have lived in the best of times as far as seeing change and I have lived in the worst of times as far as seeing my friends dying all around me. So it balances out to an extent and I am able to handle it, although at times with great emotion. It's just part of my life that I relish like a big steak after a week of being a vegetarian. So the chance to talk and search down there and pull them up is a great gift. It was the most wondrous time that I could possibly imagine.

Robin Tichane Very few people are taking the distance to step back and say "It's already 10,000 and it's certainly going to be another 25,000 in this little town." That's what artwork is for – both perceiving the inner, the invisible, as well as the big picture. That's, I think, beginning to happen with my work. It has both that inner, you know looking in, and the big picture which is kind of staggering.

David Pattent If I had a dream, it would be to have all my friends who have died to a cocktail party, to be able to sit and talk to all of those hundreds and hundreds of people that have died and just talk to them and ask them "What's your perception?" and to be able to have that reality back again and not feel that sense of loss, knowing that that person is no longer a part of the reality. They may be a part of the experience, but they're not part of the reality any more.

Peter Groubert The people I lost through the war, it's much easier to understand. They were friends and we lived together in the barracks. I knew them and knew stuff about them, but then we separated and they died. I heard about it and it was definitely a loss. But as people started dying in my community, these were people that, many of them, I had liked, loved and was very intimate with. I shared feelings with them. You know, at the beginning I was numb. As each one that died, I guess I was glad that it wasn't me and I was sad that it was them. I constantly find myself walking down the street and seeing somebody that I know and then all of a sudden I realize that they are dead and I sigh a big sigh. And I'll stop and then I'll think about something nice about them and I'll smile. It turns a feeling of emptiness into a nice memory.

My Christmas list for cards, I went over it the year before last and there were eighty names missing from my list. There are hundreds missing from my Rolodex, truly hundreds. And now there's very few people. I think maybe seven or eight that I know are still alive and I see them at the fairs and at parades. Some of them are people that were just nod and hello people on the street, acquaintances, and now we give each other big hellos and hugs sometimes 'cause we all realize that we're the end of a group, the end of an era.

When I have those feelings that I see somebody I know when I am walking and I realize that they are not alive any more, I think of something pleasant, some nice memory, I've brought them back to life, they are still around. Their life was a success. They've left many good memories behind.

Cleve Jones What did we do? Who were we? I think we were the people who created the concept of the gay community. I think we were the people who went from nothing to one. I think we took the greatest risks and probably got the greatest reward, certainly got to witness the greatest change. I'm glad I'm not your age. I would not want to be young right now. I'm glad I was born when I was born. I'm glad I got to see what I got to see. But I am very thankful I had the time I had before the epidemic.

I think the experience of the first AIDS generation for people was that we share the experience of having been a very small group who knew, at the very beginning, that what happened to us would happen to the rest of the world. That's part of it, that terrible frustration of screaming as loud as you can scream and no one can hear you. I don't think the following generation has quite had that experience. It's the total silence, a total lack of response.

Peter Groubert *Bill Kraus's name came up as Peter talked about the bathhouse controversy.* I used to date him. I have pictures of him somewhere. *Then Peter pulled out an old photo album to look at pictures of old friends.*

There's Armistead . . . This is '83. *Points out another shirtless guy in the June sun.* This is Steve Hutton. His grandfather was E. F. Hutton. "When Hutton talks, people listen." This is Peter Berlin, the famous porn star. Old boyfriends and stuff, most all of them are dead, *Peter observes matter-of-factly and, as quickly as he had said it, he turns to the next page of pictures.* Ah, this is Gayday '83 . . . There's my Mom and my Dad and there's me. My brother's old girlfriend . . . This is Gayday Parade, um, all dead . . . *Picture after picture.* I could point out lots of them there, all gone. All right, well, these are . . . *This time his voice drops and trails off as he looks.* I don't know. *Peter clears his throat as he closes the scrapbook.* I'll find Bill later. I have lots of books.

Epilogue

As HIV settles into its place beside other failures of the American political landscape such as the Civil Rights Movement and the War on Poverty, it is easy to allow it to become an abstract concept. In October 1996, the AIDS quilt Cleve dreamed up was displayed in the Capitol Mall for a last time. Stretching well over fifteen football fields, it stands ever a testament of national priorities having shifted away from handling social problems such as AIDS, such as poverty. The world's largest piece of folk art has grown too large, with too many contributors, for another complete showing (Wilson, 1996). The first generation of AIDS is over. A new generation of Americans are coming of age who were not even born when the *New York Times* first reported "Cancer Outbreaks Among Homosexuals" in 1981 (Altman, 1981) and have never known a world in which AIDS did not exist. Today, one out of every ninety-two American men aged between twenty-seven and thirty-nine has HIV ("AIDS Statistics," 1995).

The years 1995 and 1996 have seen significant progress in understanding of the immune system and the opportunistic infections that kill PWAs (Jones, 1995). And unlike the grim days of 1984, policy windows are opening which offer the opportunity to actually do something about it (Kingdon, 1984). The country appears ready to pay attention to news about HIV again. After an apologetic return in 1992, Magic Johnson stepped out of retirement in 1996 with a message for his times: "Deal with it." The same week, Dr. Anthony Fauci of NIH met with President Clinton to discuss a blueprint for closer cooperation between the Federal Government and private industry to advance the way for an AIDS vaccine (Altman, 1996A). *Newsweek* utilized Johnson's return as an opportunity to report new scientific insights about HIV as a cover story. With Magic striking a Superman pose, opening his business suit to reveal a Lakers jersey, the February 12 cover read: "New Hope for Living Longer with HIV: It's More Than Magic." "You gotta give em hope," Harvey Milk repeated.

Optimism has re-entered the battle (Ness, 1996; Snow and Hanbrook, 1996; James, 1996) and has been confirmed by reports from the 1996

Vancouver AIDS Conference (Altman, 1996D, E, F, G, H, I; Dunlap, 1996B; Dunlap and Fisher, 1996). The steps to make HIV a chronic manageable infection and discover a cure will be found if dollars are invested (Jones, 1995). With record speed, the FDA approved three new AIDS protease inhibitors early in 1996 (Hilts, 1996B; Hutchcraft, 1996). Triple drug therapies are now coming close to repressing HIV to near zero (Altman, 1996B; Susman, 1996). New insights about the route of infection and gene makeup of PWAs make further breakthroughs possible (Altman, 1996J; Leary, 1996; Maugh II, 1996).

In addition, caution, always at bay with the cancerous epidemic, remains part of the battle. Questions remain about who will be able to afford the new, by no means inexpensive, AIDS drugs (Gallagher, 1996; Cowley, 1996; Altman, 1996C; Kramer, 1996). These questions of access and equitability offer AIDS activism a way out of the *huis clos*.

As the last decade of false starts and disappointments has painfully illustrated, the new AIDS treatments must be viewed with skepticism (Rotello, 1996). Only a few years ago, it was AZT that produced this same jubilation. Many of the early tests for AZT were halted early because of the initial success in the short term. The same could be the case with protease inhibitors (Mirken, 1996).

This has not prevented the implication, created by Sullivan's (1996) "When AIDS Ends" and Leland's (1996) *Newsweek* cover story, that we have arrived at "The End of AIDS?" Autopsies, however, are premature, morally unconscionable, and even dangerous. Since the first gay men began showing up with Kaposi's Sarcoma lesions in 1980, AIDS has presented America with the greatest ethical challenge of our era. The issues it forces America to bring to bear involve strikingly familiar themes of inequality. Today, HIV disproportionately afflicts a new, almost invisible, and easy to kick around, population, the urban poor (Fullilove, 1993; Timmons, 1996; Hilts, 1996A). Suggestions that AIDS is over deem their loss insignificant; to do so implies that we've learned nothing from a decade of cries that silence is compliance.

○ ● ○ ● ○

For a while there, the minimization of leprosy, the eradication of smallpox, and the near eradication of polio demonstrated that the battle against infectious diseases appeared over. These successes reflected the possibilities of science moving us toward the eventual perfection of human life (Kurtz, 1984: 9). As the century comes to a close, however, a resurgence of infectious diseases looms. AIDS may be the tip of the iceberg (Lederberg, 1996). Seventeen million died of infectious diseases in 1995 alone (Fletcher, 1996; Butts, 1995). AIDS culminates a century of uncertainty. As the story of this disease demonstrates, our successes are always relative. And, in turn, it forces us to acknowledge the limits of science (Horgan, 1996) and policy in solving intractable problems.

The cycles of life and disease continue. Stories about disease eventually all fall into the same form. Whenever it looks like we are about to pull ourselves out, a new test returns malignant. In the end, they all become retreads of Defoe's *Journal of the Plague Year* and Camus' *The Plague*. "All we ever hear is 'so and so's dead' and 'so and so's dying' and if there were anyone left to mourn, the whole place would be filled with wailing and weeping," Boccaccio's heroines of fourteenth-century pestilent Florence complained in perhaps the first work of pure fiction, *The Decameron*. Apprehensions regarding conventional morality tend to go out the window in the face of mass carnage. Through such events we are inspired to escape from our realities to other worlds, to other tales. Boccaccio relieved his heroines by sending them out of the Church of Santa Maria Novella, where they had taken refuge, to the Tuscan country to tell stories. As stories are prone to do, they sustained them.

Early in the interview process, I talked to a man whose dementia intensified between interviews. At the end of the final interview he stopped, got up and vomited. When he sat back down he stared earnestly and told me, "Ben, if you can do anything, tell the world this isn't a joke." He died two months later. Art, Marija, Philip, Mike (and others) all died after their interviews. On Christmas Eve 1994, Fenton Johnson addressed the need for our secular culture to allow itself room to ponder the mysteries behind these deaths and lives. His call for memories of lost friends and a place for story-telling speaks a great deal for what is missing in our reified, celebrity-obsessed culture: "I remember a story of someone gone from my life, and tell it to somebody else, and in the telling of that story take my proper and necessary place in the chain of being." Through the story-telling process, the grieving, the laughing, this cycle of being, we preserve memory of the quieter voices behind this, one of the most important social histories of our time. The suffering, the lost friends behind the pandemic, are not abstract concepts. According to the World Health Organization, HIV has taken twenty million adult lives. More than a million people died last year (Fletcher, 1996). As we witness them, these voices help illuminate the concept that behind each of these deaths lived a human being with a story. Their deaths leave a huge void, a chasm.

References

AIDS Cure Act 3310 Working Group. 1994. McClintock AIDS Cure Act. ACT UP San Francisco. Dave Pasquarelli organizer.

AIDS Statistics. 1995. *The Advocate* (26 December): 12.

Alders C. T. 1993. HIV Vulnerability and the Adult Survivor of Childhood Sexual Abuse. *Child Abuse and Neglect* 17 (2) (March/April): 291–8.

Altman, Lawrence. 1981. Cancer Outbreaks Among Homosexuals. *San Francisco Chronicle* (dispatched from the *New York Times*), (3 July): A18.

Altman, Lawrence. 1996A. US-Industry Blueprint Is Drawn to Smooth the Way for An AIDS Vaccine. *New York Times* (13 February): B10 and 6.

Altman, Lawrence. 1996B. 3-Drug Therapy Shows Promise Against AIDS. *New York Times* (30 January): B6.

Altman, Lawrence. 1996C. New AIDS Therapies Arise, But Who Can Afford the Bill? *New York Times* (6 February): A1.

Altman, Lawrence. 1996D. AIDS Meeting, Signs of Hope and Obstacles. *New York Times* (6 July): A1.

Altman, Lawrence. 1996E. India Quickly Leads in H.I.V. Cases, AIDS Meeting Hears. *New York Times* (8 July): A3.

Altman, Lawrence. 1996F. At Meeting on AIDS, Experts Find Mixture of Hope and Fear. *New York Times* (9 July): B10.

Altman, Lawrence. 1996G. Powerful Response Reported To a Combined Therapy. *New York Times* (11 July): A12.

Altman, Lawrence. 1996H. Scientists Display Substantial Gains in AIDS Treatment. *New York Times* (12 July): A1 and 10.

Altman, Lawrence. 1996I. Landmark Studies Change Outlook of AIDS Treatment, New Combinations of Drugs Show Promise. *New York Times* (14 July): A10.

Altman, Lawrence. 1996J. A Discovery Energizes AIDS Researchers, Preliminary Steps Are Under Way to Explore a Genetic Mutation. *New York Times* (10 August): Y7.

Anderson, Carol M. and Stewart, Susan. 1983. *Mastering Resistance: A Practical Guide to Family Therapy*. New York: Guilford Press. P. 1.

Appletome, Peter. 1990. Dentist Dies of AIDS, Leaving Florida City Concerned but Calm. *New York Times* (8 September): A1 and 10.

Asbury, Herbert. 1933. *The Barbary Coast: An Informal History of the San Francisco Underworld*. New York: Garden City Publishing Company, Inc.

Ashley, Ronnie. 1995. Interview by author. San Francisco, CA. 29 June.

Associated Press. 1989. San Francisco Opera Debut Is Disrupted by AIDS Group, Demanding AIDS be made a top national priority. *New York Times* (10 September): A32. Certainly opera fans were already sympathetic. This disruption soured many to the cause.

Associated Press. 1995. Carrier's AIDS Fear Halts Mail to Couple. *The Arizona Republic* (14 July): A10.

Atlas, James. 1996. The Age of the Literary Memoir is Now. *New York Times Magazine* (12 May): 26.

Bay Area Report. 1993A. Shanti To Repay City Money. *San Francisco Chronicle* (5 May): A13.

Bay Area Report. 1993B. Shanti Must Repay More Misspent Money. *San Francisco Chronicle* (3 June): A22.

Bedian, Arthur and Zammuto, Raymond. 1991. *Organizations: Theory and Design*. Orlando, FL: Dryden Press: 45.

Berke, Richard L. 1996. If Clinton Sees Votes in South, He's Not Just Whistling Dixie. *New York Times* (13 September): A14. This report addresses aspects of the political capital Gays in the Military cost Clinton.

Bersani, Leo. 1991. Is the Rectum A Grave? In *AIDS: Cultural Analysis/Cultural Activism*. ed. Douglas Crimp. Boston, MA: MIT Press.

Betsey, Hazel L. 1995. Interview by author. San Francisco, CA. 30 July.

Blazer, Philip M. 1994. Interview by author. San Francisco, CA. 4 April and 2 May.

Boccaccio, Giovanni. *The Decameron*. New York: Penguin Books, 1972 edn.

Borden, William. 1991. Beneficial Outcomes in Adjustment to HIV Seropositivity. *Social Service Review* (September): 434–49.

Borden, William. 1992. Narrative Perspectives in Psychosocial Intervention Following Adverse Life Events. *Social Work* 37 (March): 135–40.

Botkin, Michael C. 1995. SF Model – R.I.P. *Bay Area Reporter* (29 June): 26.

Boulanger, Robert. 1995. Interview by author. San Francisco, CA. 6 June.

Bowlby, J. 1979. *The Making and Breaking of Affectional Bonds*. London: Tavistock Publications.

Braithwaite, Ronald L. and Lythcott, Ngina. 1991. Community Empowerment as a Strategy for Health Promotion for Black and Other Minority Populations. In *The AIDS Reader: Social, Political, Ethical Issues*. ed. Nancy F. McKenzie. New York: A Meridian Book, 524.

Braverman, G'dali. 1994. Interview by author. San Francisco, CA. 2 November.

Brodkin, Evelyn and Lipsky, Michael. 1983. Quality Control in AFDC as an Administrative Strategy. *Social Service Review* (March): 1–34.

Bronfrenbrenner, U. 1979. "Purpose and Perspective" and "Basic Concepts." In *The Ecology of Human Development*. Cambridge, MA: Harvard University Press.

Bronski, Michael. 1989. Death and the Erotic Imagination. In *Personal Dispatches: Writers Confront AIDS*. ed. John Preston. New York: St. Martin's Press.

Brown, Chip. 1995. The Experiments of Dr. Oz. *New York Times Magazine* (30 July): 21–3.

Butts, Mickey. 1995. The Coming Plague. *SF Weekly* (18 January): 22.

Cafferty, Pastora San Juan and Chestant, Leon (eds). 1976. *The Diverse Society: Implications for Public Policy*. Washington, DC.

Cailleau, John. 1994. Interview by author. San Francisco, CA. 7 and 10 May.

Carrol, Jon. 1991. One White Guy Sittin Around Rantin'. *San Francisco Chronicle* (3 July): E10. This reports on counterproductive tactical failures of AIDS activists.

Chavez, Richard. 1994. Interview by author. San Francisco, CA. 26 April.

Chew, Sally. 1993. What's Going Down at ACT UP? *Out Magazine* (October/ November). This essay features interview segments with G'dali Braverman.

Chrysler, S. 1995. AIDS Survivors Hit By Symptoms. *San Francisco Sentinel* (17 July): 17, 32, and 36.

Cohan, Gary R. 1996. Two Hats. *The Advocate* (14 May): 47.

Cohler, B. 1982. Personal Narrative and the Life Course. In P. Bates and O. Brim (eds), *Life Span Development and Human Behavior*. New York: Academic Press.

Cohler, B. 1989. Adversity, Resilience, and the Study of Lives. In E.J. Anthony and B. Cohler, *The Invulnerable Child*. New York: Guilford.

Comeau, Ray P. 1979. Night of Fire, Impressions of Bloody Monday. *Bay Area Reporter*, (7 June): 1.

Conkin, Dennis. 1994. AIDS Activists Zap Feinstein. *Bay Area Reporter* (25 August).

Cowan, David and Kuenster, John. 1996. *To Sleep with Angels: the Story of a Fire*. Chicago: Ivan R. Dee.

Cowley, Geoffrey. 1996. New Hope for Living Longer with HIV. *Newsweek* (12 February): 61–3. Cover: Its More Than Magic: 56–9.

Craiy, Gwenn. 1979. No Apologies. *Bay Area Reporter* (7 June). Craiy was the Vice-President of the Harvey Milk Gay Democratic Club. This address was given at the May 29th meeting of that club.

D'Aulaire, Ingri and Parin, Edgar. 1962. *Book of Greek Myths*. Garden City, New York: Doubleday & Company.

Dalton, Harlon L. 1991. AIDS in Blackface. In *The AIDS Reader: Social, Political, Ethical Issues*, ed. Nancy F. McKenzie. New York: A Meridian Book.

Daniels, Norman. 1995. *Seeking Fair Treatment: From the AIDS Epidemic to National Health Care Reform*. New York: Oxford University Press.

Davis, Darnell. 1994. Interview by author. San Francisco, CA. 17 September.

Denison, Rebecca. 1995. Call Us Survivors! Women Organized to Respond to Life Threatening Diseases (WORLD). In *Women Resisting AIDS: Feminist Strategies of Empowerment*, ed. Beth E. Schneider and Nancy E. Stroller. Philadelphia: Temple University Press, pp. 195–207.

Deparle, Jason. 1990. Rude, Rash, Effective, Act-Up Shifts AIDS Policy. *New York Times* (3 January): B1 and B4.

Derfler, Leslie (ed). 1990. *An Age of Conflict: Readings in Twentieth Century European History*. New York: Harcourt, Brace, Jovanovich.

Donahue, John D. 1989. *The Privatization Decision: Public Ends, Private Means*. New York: Basic Books, Inc.

Duesberg, Peter. 1996. *Inventing the AIDS Virus*. Washington: Regnery Publishing.

Dunlap, David W. 1996A. Some Gay Rights Advocates Question Effort to Defend Same-Sex Marriage. *New York Times* (7 June): A8.

Dunlap, David W. 1996B. In the AIDS Fight, Bells of Hope from Vancouver. At a Conference, Talk of Life, Not Death. *New York Times* (15 July): A6.

Dunlap, David W. and Fisher, Lawrence M. 1996. Drug Makers Get Aggressive In Pitching AIDS Treatment. *New York Times* (5 July): A1 and C6.

Earl-Keen, Robert. 1988. I Wanna Know. *The Live Album*. Durham, NC: Sugarhill Records.

Eckholm, Eric. 1994. HIV Negatives. *New York Times* (14 March): E1.

Eidspjeld, Per. 1994. Interview by author. San Francisco, CA. 25 July.

Elson, M. 1988. Kohut and Stern: Two Views of Infancy and Childhood. *Smith College Studies in Social Work*, 131–45.

Emke, Ivan. 1993. Medical Authority and Its Discontents: the Case of Organized Non-Compliance. *Critical Sociology* 19: 57–80.

Epstein, Laura. 1992. *Brief Treatment and a New Look at the Task-Centered Approach*. New York: Macmillan Publishing Company.

Epstein, Robert. 1984. *Times of Harvey Milk*. Black Sand Productions.

Ezell, Mark and Patti, Rino J. State Human Service Agencies: Structure and Organization. *Social Service Review* (March 1990).

Fandel, Michael. 1995. Interview by author. San Francisco, CA. 21 July.

Feinberg, David B. 1994. *Queer and Loathing: The Rants and Raves of a Raging AIDS Clone*. New York: Viking.

Feinstein, A. D. 1979. Personal Mythology as a Paradigm for a holistic public psychology. *American Journal of Orthopsychiatry* 49: 198–217.

Fernandez, Elizabeth. 1991. A City Responds. In *The AIDS Reader: Social, Political, Ethical Issues*, ed. Nancy F. McKenzie. New York: A Meridian Book.

Firestone, Harold. 1976. *Victims of Change: Juvenile Delinquents in American Society*. Westport, CT: Greenwood Press.

Fisher, Arthur. 1995. Interview by author. San Francisco, CA. 28 April.

Fletcher, David. 1996. Infectious Diseases Become a Global Threat. *Chicago Sun Times* (20 May): 32.

Fong-Torres, Ben. 1993. Faces of AIDS, Local Art World's Casualty List. *San Francisco Chronicle* (28 March): 25.

Ford, Dave. 1995. Eating Our Own: Infighting in the Gay Community. *S.F. Bay Times* (13 July): 3.

Franklin, Donna L. 1986. Mary Richmond and Jane Addams: From Moral Certainty to Rational Inquiry in Social Work Practice. *Social Service Review* (December): 509–10.

Freedman, Jill and Combs, Gene. 1996. *Narrative Therapy: The Social Construction of Preferred Realities.* New York: W. W. Norton.

Frumpkin *et al.* 1993. Evaluation of State Level Integration of Human Services. *Administration in Social Work* 7 (1) (Spring): 13–25.

Fullilove, Mindy Thompson. 1993. Ethnic Minorities, HIV Disease and the Growing Underclass. In *Face to Face: A Guide to AIDS Counseling,* eds James W. Dilley, Cheri Pies, and Michael Helquist. San Francisco: AIDS Health Project, 230–40.

Gallagher, John. 1996. The Money Pit. The remarkable advances reported at this year's international AIDS conference may be too costly to help most people with HIV. *The Advocate* (3 September): 29–30.

Garfield, Charles (ed.). 1978. *Psychological Care and the Dying Patient.* New York: McGraw-Hill.

Garfield, Charles (ed.). 1995. *Sometimes My Heart Goes Numb.* San Francisco: Jossey-Bass.

Garfield, Charles A. and Clark, Rachel Ogren. 1978. The Shanti Project: A Community Model. *Death Education* (Winter): 397–408.

Garfield, Charles A. and Spring, Cindy. 1993. *AIDS Caregiving: Lessons for the Second Decade.* San Francisco: Jossey-Bass.

Gay, Peter. 1968. *Weimar Culture.* Westport, CT: Greenwood Press.

Gay, Peter. 1988. *Freud: A Life for Our Time.* New York: W. W. Norton.

Germain, C. B. 1990. Life Forces and the Anatomy of Practice. *Smith College Studies in Social Work* 60 (2): 138–52.

Ghez, Marissa. 1995. Communications & Public Education: Effective Tools to Promote Cultural Change. Presented at the Violence Against Women Strategic Planning Meeting. National Institute of Justice. Washington, DC. March 31.

Gilbert, Susan. 1995. Doctors Often Fail to Heed the Wishes of the Dying Patient. *New York Times* (22 November): A1 and B12.

Gitlin, Todd. 1995. *The Twilight of Common Dreams: Why America is Wracked by Culture Wars.* New York: Henry Holt and Company.

Gluck, Robert. 1989. HTLV-3. In *Personal Dispatches: Writers Confront AIDS,* ed. John Preston. New York: St. Martin's Press.

Goldstein, Howard. 1990. Knowledge Base in the Social Work Practice: Theory, Wisdom, Analogue, or Art? *Families in Society* (January): 32–43.

Greenbaum, Paul D. 1994. Interview by author. San Francisco, CA. 14 and 21 June.

Gross, Jane. 1993. Second Wave of AIDS Feared by Officials in San Francisco. *New York Times* (11 December): 1.

Grossman, A. H. and Silverstein, C. 1993. Facilitating Support Groups for Professionals Working with People with AIDS. *Social Work* 38 (March): 145–51.

Grothe, T. and McKusick, L. 1993. Coping with Multiple Loss. In *Face to Face: A Guide to AIDS Counseling,* eds James W. Dilley, Cheri Pies, and Michael Helquist. San Francisco: AIDS Health Project, 376–9.

Groubert, Peter S. 1994. Interview by author. San Francisco, CA. 20 July.

Hartt, Frederick. 1987. *Italian Renaissance Art: Painting, Sculpture, Architecture.* New York: Harry N. Abrams.

Heale, M. J. 1990. *American Anticommunism: Combating the Enemy Within 1930–1970.* Baltimore: Johns Hopkins University Press.

Health. 1996. Unsigned. Reports from the medical front. *The Advocate* (17 September): 20.

Helminak, Daniel. 1994. *What the Bible Really Says About Homosexuality, Top Scholars Put Homosexuality in*

Perspective. San Francisco: Alamo Square Press.

Hillman, James. 1983. *Healing Fiction*. Barrytown, NY: Station Hill Press.

Hilts, Philip. 1990. $2.9 Billion Bill For AIDS Relief Gains in Senate. *New York Times* (16 May): A1 and 24.

Hilts, Philip. 1996A. AIDS Death Rate Rising in 25–44 Age Group. *New York Times* (16 February): A10.

Hilts, Philip. 1996B. With Record Speed, F.D.A. Approves a New AIDS Drug. *New York Times* (15 March): A9.

Hogan, John. 1986. *The End of Science: Facing the Limits of Knowledge in the Twilight of the Scientific Age*. Reading, MA: Addison-Wesley.

Hutchcraft, Chuck. 1996. New Clue on AIDS. *Chicago Tribune* (21 April): Section 5, p. 1.

Jacobs, Joanne. 1995. Jesse Helms Didn't Intend the Irony. *Dallas Morning News* (13 July): 21A. Also see: Associated Press. Helms Blasts Gays on Senate Floor. *San Francisco Sentinel* (26 July): 3 and 9.

James, John S. 1996. New Optimism on Controlling HIV Infection. *San Francisco Bay Times* (27 June): 343.

Ji-Ahnte, Anthony and Denise. 1994. Medical Repression. *Z Magazine* (7 May): 17–20.

Johanns, Willi. 1992. Out of the Dark: Crime, Mystery, and Suspense in German Cinema, 1915–1951. Idea, conception, and research. A film-retrospective and exhibition of the Goethe-Institute in the USA and Canada. Program.

Johnson, Fenton. 1994. Death Into Life. *New York Times* (24 December): A15.

Jones, Cleve. 1995. Priority Number One. Unpublished essay.

Jones, Cleve. 1995. Interview by author. San Francisco and Gernville, CA. 22 May and 25 August.

Jones, Cynora. 1995. Interview by author. Oakland, CA. 20 July.

Jung, Carl. 1933. *Modern Man in Search of a Soul*. New York: Harcourt, Brace & World.

Jung, Carl. 1966. *The Spirit in Man, Art, and Literature*. Princeton, NJ: Princeton University Press.

Kaes *et al.* 1994. *The Weimar Republic Sourcebook*. Berkeley, CA: The University of California Press.

Kaiser, John. 1993. *Immune Power*. New York: St. Martin's Press.

Kelley, Patricia. 1995. Integrating Narrative Approaches Into the Clinical Curricula: Addressing Diversity through Understanding. *Journal of Social Work Education* 31 (3) (Fall): 347–57.

Kierkegaard, Søren. 1859. On Himself. In *Existentialism: from Dostoevsky to Sartre*, ed. Walter Kaufmann. 1956. New York: Meridian Books.

Kingdon, John W. 1984. *Agendas, Alternatives, and Public Policies*. Boston: Little, Brown, and Company.

Kissinger, Henry, A. 1995. With Faint Praise: A Biographer Finds Traces of Clay on the Great Statesman's Feet. Review of *Churchill: The Unruly Giant*, by Norman Rose. *New York Times Book Review* (16 July): 7.

Knuckles, Yvonne. 1995. Interview by author. Oakland, CA. 20 July.

Kolata, Gina. 1995. New AIDS Findings on Why Drugs Fail, Long Immune System Battle May Alter Research Path. *New York Times* (12 January): A1.

Kramer, Larry. 1993A. Playboy Interview: Larry Kramer: a candid conversation with the angry writer and activist about love and sex, gays and straights, life and death – and politics – in the age of AIDS. Interview with David Nimmons. *Playboy* (April): 61–74.

Kramer, Larry. 1993B. We Can Do It. *The Advocate* (August): 80.

Kramer, Larry. 1996. A Good News, Bad News AIDS Joke. Finally there are drugs that may allow people to live longer, but here's the punch line: Few can afford them. *New York Times Magazine* (14 July): 26–9.

Kreiger, Lisa M. 1996. AIDSWEEK - The Toll. *San Francisco Examiner*, (26 June): p. A2.

Kris, E. 1956. The Personal Myth: A Problem in Psychoanalytic Technique.

Journal of the American Psychoanalytic Association 4: 653–81.

Krutz, Lester R. 1984. *Evaluating Chicago Sociology: A Guide to the Literature with an Annotated Bibliography.* Chicago: University of Chicago Press.

Kübler-Ross, Elizabeth. 1969. *On Death & Dying.* New York: Macmillan.

Kübler-Ross, Elizabeth. 1987. *AIDS: The Ultimate Challenge.* New York: Macmillan.

Lazarous, R. and Folkman, S. 1984. *Stress, Appraisal, and Coping.* New York: Springer.

Leary, Warren. 1996. Scientists Find Elusive Protein, H.I.V.'s Guide. *New York Times* (10 May): A1.

Lederberg, Joshua. 1996. The Flu's Lethal Future. *New York Times* (27 January): A15.

Lee, Henry K. 1996. Shanti Wins Big Judgment, Accounting Agency to Pay Agency $712,000. *San Francisco Chronicle* (9 July): A13.

Lee, Robert E. 1994. Interview by author. San Francisco, CA. 13 July.

Lehrman, Sally. 1994. City AIDS Care Net Reported Collapsing: Task Force Warns Exploding Caseload, Long-term Care, Lack of Funds Taxing National Model. *San Francisco Examiner* (1 December): A12.

Leland, John. 1996. The End of AIDS? *Newsweek* (2 December): 64.

Lemoins, Nancy. 1995. Interview by author. San Francisco, CA. 25 and 28 July.

Levinson, Daniel. 1978. *The Seasons of a Man's Life.* New York: Ballantine Books.

Lewin, Tamar. 1996. Ignoring "Right to Die" Directives, Medical Community is Being Sued. *New York Times* (2 June): A1.

Lind, Michael. 1996. Return of the Liberal: E. J. Dionne has bad news for the Republicans, but it's not necessarily good news for the Democrats. Review of *They Only Look Dead: Why Progressives Will Dominate the Next Political Era*, by E. J. Dionne. *New York Times Book Review* (18 February): 10.

Lipski, Michael. 1980. *Street-Level Bureaucracy.* New York: Russell Sage Foundation.

Lorch, P. 1979. Viewpoint: The Afterburn. *Bay Area Reporter* (7 June).

McAdams, Dan. 1990. Unity and Purpose in Human Lives: The Emergence of Identity as a Life Story. *Studying Persons and Lives*, ed. Rubin *et al.* New York: Springer, 148–52.

McDaniel, Antonio and London, Andrew S. 1995. HIV Morality and the African American Population. *National Journal of Sociology* 9.1 (Summer): 84–7.

McKenzie, Nancy F. 1991. Introduction. In *The AIDS Reader: Social, Political, Ethical Issues*, ed. Nancy F. McKenzie. New York: A Meridian Book, 1–9.

McLarty, Scott. 1994. United We Stand; Divided We Grovel: Queers and the Health Care Debate. *Z Magazine* (December): 39–40.

McNeill, William. 1976. *Plagues and Peoples.* Garden City, New York: Anchor Press/Doubleday.

McNight, John. 1987. Regenerating Community. *Social Policy* (Winter): 54–8.

Manzo, Hugo. 1995. Interview by author. San Francisco, CA. 5 July.

Marcuse, Herbert. 1964. *One Dimensional Man: Studies in the Ideology of Advanced Industrial Society.* Boston: Beacon Press.

Marcuse, Herbert. 1977. *The Aesthetic Dimension: Toward a Critique of Marxist Aesthetics.* Boston: Beacon Press.

Martin, Gerald. 1995. *Journeys Through the Labyrinth: Latin American Fiction in the Twentieth Century.* London: Verso.

Martin, Ruth R. 1995. *Oral History in Social Work: Research, Assessment and Intervention.* London: Sage Publications.

Martinez, Gabriel. 1995. Interview by author. San Francisco, CA. 1 June.

Maugh II, Thomas H. 1996. HIV Infection "Gateway" Found, Promises Fresh Approach to Treating AIDS. *Chicago Sun-Times* (20 June): 3.

Meyer, John and Rowan, Brian. 1977. Institutionalized Organizations: Formal Structure as Myth and Ceremony. *American Journal of Sociology* Vol. 83, No. 2. pp. 340–63.

Milano, Mark. 1995. Why Not a Cure? ACT UP's AIDS Cure Project will work. *POZ Magazine* (April/May): 38.

Mirken, Bruce. 1994. The state of AIDS: a Bay Area roundtable. *S.F. Frontiers* (18 August): 18.

Mirken, Bruce. 1995. Patient, Heal Thyself. Review of *Good Doctors, Good Patients: Partners in HIV Treatment,* by Judith Rabkin, Robert Remien, and Christopher Wilson. *Windy City Times* (7 September): 14.

Mirken, Bruce. 1996. The New AIDS Drugs. *Windy City Times* (25 April): 13.

Moller, David Wendell. 1995. *Confronting Death: Values, Institutions, and Human Mortality.* New York: Oxford University Press.

Moore, Teresa. 1993A. Shanti Gives Up $1.9 Million in Housing Contracts, Groups Board Goes Along with Recommendation. *San Francisco Chronicle* (5 July): A14.

Moore, Teresa. 1993B. Shanti Project's Director Quitting For Job In Seattle. *San Francisco Chronicle* (4 August): A16.

Morten, Frederic. 1979. *A Nervous Splendor: Vienna 1888/1889.* New York: Penguin.

Moss, J. Jennings. 1997. The Odd Couple: The fate of gay civil rights legislation could hang on the surprising alliance of two powerful and distinctly different Republican leaders. *The Advocate* (4 February), 41.

Moynihan *et al.* 1988. AIDS and Terminal Illness. *Social Casework* (June): 69, 380–7.

Mrdjenovic, Marija. 1994. Interview by author. San Francisco, CA. 19 July.

Murray, Stephen O. and Paine, Kenneth W. 1988. Medical Policy Without Scientific Evidence: The Promiscuity Paradigm of AIDS. *California Sociologist* 11 (Winter/Summer): 13–14.

Nack, William, and Munson, Lester. 1995. Sports' Dirty Little Secret. *Sports Illustrated* (31 July): 62–74.

NAPA, National Academy of Public Administration. 1977. *Reorganization in Florida: How is Services Integration Working?* Washington, DC: National Academy of Public Administration.

Neff, Jeff. 1996. Study Finds Gay Arousal in Homophobic Men. *Windy City Times* (22 August): 1 and 8. They cite a study by University of Georgia Professor Henry Adams published in *The Journal of Abnormal Psychiatry.*

Nelson, Barbara J. 1984. *Making an Issue of Child Abuse: Political Agenda Setting for Social Problems.* Chicago: University of Chicago Press.

Ness, Carol. 1996. AIDS: A Message of Hope, But the Epidemic: 42% of S.F. Gay Men Are Believed to be Infected, Fifth of Seven Part Series: Gay in America: 1996. *San Francisco Examiner* (27 June): A1, A10–11.

Neugenebauer *et al.* 1992. Bereavement Reactions Among Homosexual Men Experiencing Multiple Losses in the AIDS Epidemic. *American Journal of Psychiatry* (October): 149, 1374–9.

Nuland, Sherwin B. 1994. *How We Die: Reflections on Life's Final Chapter.* New York: A. A. Knopf.

Null, Gary, PhD. 1995. HIV Equals AIDS and Other Myths of the AIDS War. *Penthouse* (December): 118.

O'Brien, Tim. 1994. Back to My Lai: A Fractured Love Story. *New York Times Magazine* (2 October).

Odets, Walt. 1995. The Fatal Mistakes of AIDS Education. *San Francisco Bay Times* (4 May): 3–7. Essay based on Odets' at the time upcoming work *In the Shadow of the Epidemic: Being HIV Negative In the Age of AIDS* (1996), Duke University Press. (Interviews with Odets are in Jessee Green (1996) Just Say No? When public health campaigns try to change private behavior, they rarely work – and the failure of the safe-sex message to reach men like Mark Ebenhock shows why. *The New York Times Magazine* (15 September).)

Pae, Mi Young. 1994. Shanti Project Moves, Celebrates 20 Years in Health Service. *San Francisco Chronicle* (29 June): D3.

Parsons, Talcott. 1951. *The Social System.* New York: The Free Press.

Pattent, David. 1994. Interview by author. San Francisco, CA. 8 October.

Perrow, Charles. 1978. Demystifying Organizations. In *The Management of Human Services*, ed. Sarri and Hasenfeld. New York: Columbia University Press, 105–23.

Petit, Bruce. 1979A. Do "Good People" Plan Murder? White's All-Hetero Jury Weighs Premeditation. *Bay Area Reporter* (10 May): 1.

Petit, Bruce. 1979B. Gays Explode at Manslaughter, Non-Gays Join More Violent Second Phase. *Bay Area Reporter* (24 May): 1. The unsigned cover story read: Gays Riot: WHY – WHY NOT?

Petit, Bruce. 1979C. White's Guilt: Obvious Yet Complex. *Bay Area Reporter* (24 May): 5.

Phillips, Adam. 1994. The Telling of the Self. In *On Flirtation.* Cambridge, MA: Harvard University Press.

Plummer, Ken. 1983. *Documents of Life: An Introduction to the Problems and Literature of a Humanistic Method.* London: George Allen & Unwin Ltd.

Pollack, Andrew. 1994. Meeting Lays Bare the Abyss Between AIDS and Its Cure. *New York Times* (12 August): A1 and A6.

Posner, Joel. 1994. Interview by author. San Francisco, CA. 26 April and 3 May.

Project Inform. 1994. Unsigned Discussion Paper #3, Doctor, Patient and HIV: Building a Cooperative Relationship.

Provenzano, Jim. 1993. Shanti Holds Open Forum Tonight. *Bay Area Reporter* (28 October): 1.

Purnell, Rogéair Damone. 1996. "Child Sexual Abuse, Alcohol and Drug (Mis)Use, Among African-American Women: An Exploratory Study." A presentation at the University of Chicago School of Social Service Administration to the Faculty Search Committee (11 March).

Radosh, Ronald. 1996. *Divided They Fell: The Demise of the Democratic Party 1964–96.* New York: The Free Press.

Raine, George and Flinn, John. 1994. 2,000 Salute Shilts' Efforts in AIDS Assault. *San Francisco Examiner* (23 February): A4.

Reid, William J. 1992. *Task Strategies: An Empirical Approach to Clinical Social Work.* New York: Columbia University Press.

Reuters. 1995. Early Use of AIDS Drug Is Termed Not Effective. *New York Times* (17 August): A10.

Reyes, Marcos. 1995. Interview by author. San Francisco, CA. 6 June.

Rich, Frank. 1995. Dance of Death. *New York Times* (8 January): A15.

Riessman, Catherine Kohler. 1993. *Narrative Analysis: Qualitative Research Methods* Volume Methods Series, Vol. 30. Newbury Park: Sage.

Roberts, Jerry. 1994. White Knight. In *Never Let Them See You Cry: A Biography of Diane Feinstein.* San Francisco: Harper Collins West, 185–9.

Rofes, Eric. 1996. *Reviving the Tribe: Regenerating Gay Man's Sexuality and Culture in the Ongoing Epidemic.* Birmingham, NY: Harrington Park Press.

Rojas, Todd. 1994. Shanti Must Pay Refund to SF Book Keepers Blamed for Problems, Declining Donations Noted. *San Francisco Chronicle* (5 January): A15.

Rotello, Gabrielle. 1996. The Risk in a "Cure" For AIDS. *New York Times* (14 July): E17.

Rottkamp, Russell. 1995. Hope, Anger Aired at Project Inform Dinner. *San Francisco Sentinel* (10 May): 3.

Rubin, Allen and Babbie, Earl. 1993. *Research Methods for Social Work.* Pacific Grove, CA.: Brooks Cole Publishing Company.

Sabin, Russell. 1992. AIDS Charity Offers Housing for Sufferers. Shanti Project Renovated a 65-Unit Apartment Building. *San Francisco Chronicle* (5 December): A20.

Sabin, Russell. 1993A. Audit of Shanti Find Problems. $200,000 May Have Gone to Worthy But Unauthorized Projects. *San Francisco Chronicle* (10 March): A11.

Sabin, Russell. 1993B. Shanti Project Admits It May Owe $310,000 in Overpayments. *San Francisco Chronicle* (4 May): A15.

San Francisco Chronicle. 1979. F.B.I. Probes Police Riot. *Bay Area Reporter* (19 July): 1. This report was first run in the *Chronicle* and then picked up by the *BAR*.

Schlesinger, Arthur. 1996. History as Therapy: A Dangerous Idea. *New York Times* (3 May): A11.

Schmalz, Jeffrey. 1993. What Ever Happened to AIDS? *New York Times Magazine* (28 November): 86.

Schmitt, Eric. 1996. President Plans to Sign Bill to Cut Troops with H.I.V. *New York Times* (27 January): A6.

Second Wave, The. 1995. Hamlin, John. *60 Minutes*, CBS (9 April).

Segal, Jay. 1994. Interview by author. San Francisco, CA. 30 April.

Sentinel, The. 1978. Thousands March In Silent Tribute. Unsigned Story. *The Sentinel* (1 December): 7. Also see: In Memoriam: Slain Leaders Laid To Rest As Thousands Pay Tribute: 1.

Shaw, Clifford. 1931. *The Natural History of Delinquent Career* Chicago: University of Chicago Press.

Shaw, Nancy Stoller. 1991. Preventing AIDS Among Women: The Role of Community Organizing. In *The AIDS Reader: Social, Political, Ethical Issues*, ed. Nancy F. McKenzie. New York: A Meridian Book: 504–21.

Shaw, Nancy Stoller. 1993. HIV Disease: Issues for Women. In *Face to Face: A Guide to AIDS Counseling*, eds James W. Dilley, Cheri Pies, and Michael Helquist. San Francisco: AIDS Health Project, 241–8.

Shepard, Ben. 1994A. Bodies as Billboards: Tee Shirt Designer and Veteran of '70s Castro, John Cailleau. *Bay Area Reporter* (16 June): 78.

Shepard, Ben. 1994B. Looking In, Not At: A Chat with Robin Tichane. *Bay Area Reporter* (21 July): 45.

Shepard, Ben. 1995. Maria. *Antioch Review* (Spring): 156–68.

Shepard, Ben. 1996. Choosing Their Battles. *Minnesota Review* (Spring): 35–49.

Shepnick, Philippe. 1995. ACT UP's split over issues. *San Francisco Sentinel* (26 July): 1 and 6.

Sherbert, Brad. 1995. Interview by author. San Francisco, CA. 20 June.

Sherman, Edmund, and Reid, William J. 1994. *Qualitative Research in Social Work*. New York: Columbia University Press.

Shilts, Randy. 1982. *The Mayor of Castro Street: The Life and Times of Harvey Milk.* New York: St. Martin's Press.

Shilts, Randy. 1987. *And the Band Played On.* New York: St. Martin's Press.

Shilts, Randy. 1992. Foreword. In Pogash, Carol, *As Real as It Gets: The Life of a Hospital at the Center of the AIDS Epidemic*. New York: Plume, xi.

Shilts, Randy. 1994. Interview by Michael H. Bravshow. *60 Minutes*, CBS (17 July).

Simmons, Todd. 1995. Living on the Edge. *The Advocate* (26 December): 25–8.

Skocpol, Theda. 1996. *Boomerang: Clinton's Health Security Effort and the Turn Against Government in U.S. Politics*. New York: W. W. Norton.

Snow, Bill and Hanbrook, Larry. ACT UP Writers Pool. 1996. New Options For New Infections. *Bay Area Reporter* (20 June): 20.

Sosin, Michael R. 1990. Decentralizing the Social Service System: A Reassessment. *Social Service Review* (December).

Stanger, Mark E. 1994. Interview by author. San Francisco, CA. 19 October.

Stein, George and Plimpton, George. 1982. *Eddie: An American Biography*. New York: Dell.

Stryker, Susan and Buskirk, Jim Van. 1996. *Gay By the Bay: A History of Queer Culture in the San Francisco Bay Area*. San Francisco: Chronicle Books.

Sullivan, Andrew. 1996. When AIDS Ends. *New York Times Magazine* (18 November).

SUPPORT. 1995. A Controlled Trial to Improve Care for Seriously Ill Hospitalized Patients. The Study to Understand and Preferences for

Outcomes and Risks of Treatments (SUPPORT). *Journal of the American Medical Association* 274 (22/29 November): 1591–8.

Susman Ed. 1996. Multidrug Use Suppresses HIV in the Long-Term. Is Quadruple-Therapy the Next Big Thing? *Bay Area Reporter* (20 June): 21.

Swenson, Robert M. 1988. Plagues, History, and AIDS. *The American Scholar* (Spring): 183–200.

Swissler, Mary Ann and Salinas, Mike. 1995. Kramer, Fauci Speak and Get Zapped at Project Inform Dinner. *Bay Area Reporter* (11 May): 14–15.

Terkel, Studs. 1967. *Division Street: America*. New York: Avon Books.

Thomas, R. E. 1994. Interview by author. San Francisco, CA. 20 April.

Tuller, David. 1993. Uninfected Gays Suffering, Too. *San Francisco Chronicle* (19 March): A1.

Tichane, Robin. 1993. *AIDS: Dark Terrain*. Handmade book. San Francisco.

Tichane, Robin. 1994. Interview by author. San Francisco, CA. 27 and 29 June.

Timmons, Stuart. 1996. Blood and Money. *Vibe* (August): 98–104.

Tracking the AIDS Economy. 1995. Unsigned report. *San Francisco Frontiers* (11 May): 8–21. Included in this report is the essay, Cash Crunch: Trials and Tribulations of Bay Area AIDS Fundraising, by Bruce Mirken. The essay features an interview with G'dali Braverman.

Trattner, Walter I. 1994. *From Poor Law To Welfare State*, 5th edn. New York: The Free Press.

Treatment Strategy, Project Inform Discussion Paper #1, 1993. Day One . . . After You've Tested Positive. (17 May).

Truxler, Allan. 1989. Wandering the Woods in the Season of Death. In *Personal Dispatches: Writers Confront AIDS*, ed. John Preston. New York: St. Martin's Press: 43.

Verghese, Abraham. 1995. Do You Believe in Magic? Two New Books Make Case for the Existence of Miracles. Review of *Spontaneous Healing* by Andrew Weil and *Expect a Miracle: The Miracles that Happen to Ordinary People* by Dan Wakefield. *New York Times Book Review* (28 May): 22.

Vojir, Daniel. 1994. Interview by author. San Francisco, CA. 20 and 22 June.

Waldholz, Michael. 1996. Precious Pills, New AIDS Treatment Raises Tough Question of Who Will Get It, For the Poor, High Costs, Rigid Regimens, Dim Drug Cocktails Promise – A Major Issue for Medicare. *Wall Street Journal* (3 July): A1 and A12.

Weiners, Brad. 1995. Escape to San Francisco: The Books to Read if You Want to Know the Cool, Gray City of Love. *The Bay Guardian Lit.* (June): 10.

Weir, John, 1995. Blood Simple. *Details* (October): 136–8.

Weiss, Mike. 1984. *The Doubleplay: the San Francisco City Hall Killings*. Reading, MA: Addison-Wesley.

Weitman, Wendy. 1992. A Disturbing Reality: The Prints of Max Beckman. *MOMA, Max Beckman Prints from the Museum of Modern Art*. New York: Harry N. Abrams, 5–21.

White, M. and Epston, D. 1990. *Narrative Means to Therapeutic Ends*. New York: W. W. Norton.

Willet, John. 1978. *The New Sobriety: Art and Politics in the Weimar Period*. London: Thames and Hudson.

Williams, L. Rearce (ed.). 1968. *Relativity Theory: Its Origins and Impact on Modern Thought*. Malibar, FL: Robert E. Krieger Publishing Co.

Wilson, Henry "Hank." 1995. Interview by author. San Francisco, CA. 14 June.

Wilson, Terry. 1996. Stitching Against Time, Survivors Scramble to Add to AIDS Quilt. *Chicago Tribune* (26 May): Sec 4, p. 1.

Zachary, Bohdan. 1995. Winning The War. A final interview with Paul Monette. *The Advocate* (21 March): 60.

Zastrow, Charles and Ashman, Karen Kirst. 1995. *Understanding Human Behavior in the Social Environment*. Chicago: Nelson-Hall Publishers.

Index of Names

Note: entries in *italic* denote interviewees.